TECHNICAL COLLEGE OF THE LOWCOUNTRY
LEARNING RESOURCES CENTER 027709
P. O. BOX 1288
100 S. RIBAUT ROAD
BEAUFORT, S. C. 29901

Noise Control Manual

Guidelines for Problem-Solving in the
Industrial / Commercial Acoustical Environment

Edited by
David A. Harris

Sponsored by the Noise Control Association (NCA)

A NOT FOR PROFIT Association of Noise Control Products, Materials & Systems Manufacturers

VNR VAN NOSTRAND REINHOLD
_____ New York

Copyright © 1991 by Van Nostrand Reinhold

Library of Congress Catalog Card Number 91-22223
ISBN 0-442-00851-1

All rights reserved. No part of this work covered by the copyright hereon may be reproduced or used in any form or by any means—graphic, electronic, or mechanical, including photocopying, recording, taping, or informaton storage and retrieval systems—without written permission of the publisher.

Manufactured in the United States of America

Published by Van Nostrand Reinhold
115 Fifth Avenue
New York, New York 10003

Chapman and Hall
2-6 Boundary Row
London, SE1 8HN, England

Thomas Nelson Australia
102 Dodds Street
South Melbourne 3205
Victoria, Australia

Nelson Canada
1120 Birchmount Road
Scarborough, Ontario M1K 5G4, Canada

16 15 14 13 12 11 10 9 8 7 6 5 4 3 2 1

Library of Congress Cataloging-in-Publication Data

Noise control manual : guidelines for problem-solving in the industrial/commercial acoustical environment / edited by David A. Harris
   p. cm.
  Includes bibliographical references and index.
  ISBN 0-442-00851-1
  1. Noise control   I. Harris, David A., 1934-   .
TD892.N6537   1991
620.2'3--dc20
                                            91-22223
                                              CIP

CONTENTS

Preface	v
Acknowledgments	vii
Chapter 1 - NOISE CONTROL TECHNOLOGY	1
Chapter 2 - MATERIALS FOR NOISE CONTROL	9
Chapter 3 - SOUND BARRIER MATERIALS/SYSTEMS	23
Chapter 4 - VIBRATION DAMPING MATERIALS	35
Chapter 5 - SILENCERS	45
Chapter 6 - VIBRATION ISOLATION MATERIALS	53
Chapter 7 - SYSTEMS FOR NOISE CONTROL	63
Chapter 8 - OFFICE ACOUSTICS	81
Appendix 1 - GLOSSARY OF ACOUSTICAL TERMS	95
Appendix 2 - ACOUSTICAL STANDARDS	101

Appendix 3 - DESIGN GUIDE and WORKSHEETS
    dB_A Calculations
    Guidelines for Reverberant Noise Control
    Worksheet for Reverberant Noise Control
    Source, Path and Receiver Control (SPR)
    Sound Attenuation Nomogram
    Controlling Noise at Receiver
    Controlling Environmental Noise
	119

Appendix 4 - ACOUSTICAL DATA	141
Appendix 5 - BIBLIOGRAPHY and INDEX	157, 159

PREFACE

Excessive noise levels are generally acknowledged to have adverse effects on our environment. Studies indicate that excessive noise levels can cause fatigue in exposed individuals, lower efficiency and productivity, impaired speech communication, and hearing loss. Excessive noise is almost everywhere today - in the office, in schools, hospitals and other institutional facilities, in all classes of public buildings, and in our factories.

INDUSTRIAL NOISE

High noise levels in factories can make speech communication in the plant difficult and at times impossible. Foremen are often unable to hear warning shouts from co-workers.

The problem of hearing loss due to excessive noise exposure is of particular concern to industry, and to the federal government. In the early 1970s, the United States Congress passed the Occupational Safety and Health Act (OSHA) which sets criteria for health hazards and established limits for noise exposure of industrial workers. The OSHA Noise Standard was amended in 1982 to require audiometric testing of all employees exposed to noise levels of 85 dB_A or above for eight hours.

NOISE IN COMMERCIAL AND INSTITUTIONAL BUILDINGS

While noise levels in offices, stores, schools, and other commercial and institutional buildings seldom reach those encountered in many industrial environments, they often reach levels which are distracting to the occupants of such buildings. Impairment of speech communication among workers, or inversely the lack of speech privacy, are both deterrents to efficiency and productivity and are detrimental to the occupants' comfort and sense of well-being.

The noise problem can be particularly troublesome in the increasingly used open office environment, where the efficiencies and cost benefits of this space use concept may be largely negated without careful and professional attention to the acoustical properties of the space.

THE PROBLEM EXTENDS OUTSIDE THE PLANT

Excessive noise levels are often experienced by individuals beyond plant boundaries. Nearby residents, office personnel, and visitors to noisy plants are often similarly exposed to excessive noise and are likewise subject to the adverse effects of such noise on health and well-being.

In such cases, especially when noisy plants or airports are located adjacent to residential areas, community relations problems arise. Often, such facilities are in violation of local codes governing noise.

Due to concern over excessive noise levels in our environment, the Environmental Protection Agency (EPA) has legislated noise levels in certain industries. For example, the transportation industry has established specific guidelines for manufacturers which limit the allowable noise produced by heavy trucks.

THE PROBLEM HAS ANSWERS

The problems of hearing impairment, of lessened employee productivity and morale, of diminished worker health, and of community action arising as a result of excessive noise emissions, can be effectively reduced or eliminated by proper acoustical treatments. Most noise control problems can be resolved by one or more of the following:

- Treating the **source** of the noise, either by mechanical corrective action or by application of acoustical material.
- Treating the **path** taken by noise as it travels directly and/or via reflecting routes from the source to the listener.
- Treating the **receiver** (i.e., the position of the listener) by constructing an acoustically efficient enclosure.

Often, a combination of these three treatments may be required.

NCA SOLUTIONS TO NOISE CONTROL PROBLEMS

NCA members manufacture a wide range of products that can be effectively employed to reduce excessive noise levels. This manual contains descriptions of a variety of these products, provides specific examples of their use, and includes acoustical values for these products derived from laboratory tests. With this information, plus the brief and practical approach to understanding and controlling noise presented in this brochure, engineers should be able to deal effectively and economically with many sound control problems.

ACKNOWLEDGMENTS

The NOISE CONTROL ASSOCIATION (NCA) sponsored the preparation of this manual with the intent to provide appropriate technical information about noise control technology, materials, products, systems, testing and problem solving techniques. NCA is a **not for profit** Association of noise control products, materials and systems manufacturers. NCA was renamed in 1989; the prior name was Noise Control Products and Materials Association (NCPMA).

The OBJECTIVES of NCA are to:

- Cooperate for the improvement of the industry.
- Sponsor programs directed towards the further development of business for all members of the industry.
- Educate present and future noise control users to increase the market potential for the industry.
- Establish and utilize liaisons with other associations, government agencies, and educational institutions.
- Cooperate in the development of voluntary consensus standards with related organizations.
- Serve as a focal point for all who want to make contact with the industry.
- Serve as a coordinating and implementing factor, that those in the noise control industry may combine their talents, experience, and resources to work on solutions to mutual problems.

It is the sincere hope of NCA members and the contributing authors that this manual will help the newcomer to the industry to understand basics, and will provide a reference for the experienced noise control specifier. Reasonable care has been taken to accurately include all relevant information. But because of variations in construction techniques, importance of proper installation, and other factors, neither NCA, its members or contributing authors can assume liability for results obtained by the use of this information.

Original drafts of this Noise Control Manual were produced by NCA under the direction of the Members with supervision from the Board of Directors. Many individuals participated in the preparation of this material, including current and past officers, committee chairman, and members at large. Mr. Lew Bell, consultant provided an independent review. Portions of this document were provided by Sound and Vibration Magazine from a series of articles authored by W. Earnest Purcell. Additional material is from a document authored by D. A. Harris, published by Owens Corning Fiberglas. This manual was edited by D. A. Harris, the Executive Director if the NCA. To facilitate publication, full rights of authorship and editing were assigned to David A. Harris, Principal, Building and Acoustic Design Consultants, 104 Cresta Verde Dr., Rolling Hills Est., CA 90274, (213) 377-9958.

NCA OFFICERS - 1991

PRESIDENT (3rd term)
    John W. Flood, Vice President
    ECKEL INDUSTRIES, INC., Acoustics Div.
    155 Fawcett Street
    Cambridge, MA 02138
    (617) 491-3221, FAX (617) 547-2171

VICE PRESIDENT
    Kenneth W. Kubofcik, President
    THE BRANFORD COMPANIES
    P. O. Box 713
    Shelton, CT 06489
    (203) 735-6415, FAX (203) 736-9102

SECRETARY/TREASURER
    Peter Jackson, Dir. of Tech. Services
    PERSTORP COMPONENTS - Antiphon
    2655 Woodward Ave. Suite 350
    Bloomfield Hills, MI 48013
    (313) 332-0267 FAX (313) 332-0106

DIRECTORS
    Larrie Reese, Vice President
    ILLBRUCK, INC.
    3800 Washington Ave. N.
    Minneapolis, MN 55412
    (612) 521-3555

    Robert Prybutok, President
    POLYMER TECHNOLOGIES, INC.
    7006 Pencader Drive
    Newark, DE 19702
    (302) 738-9001 FAX (302) 738-9085

    Carl Wolaver, Market Manager
    THE SOUNDCOAT COMPANY
    1 Burt Drive
    Deer Park, NY 11729, (516) 242-2200

EXECUTIVE DIRECTOR
    David A. Harris, Principal
    BLDG. & ACOUSTIC DESIGN CSLTS.
    104 Cresta Verde Drive
    Rolling Hills Est., CA 90274
    FAX & Phone: (213) 377-9958

NCA MEMBERS

THE BRANFORD COMPANIES
P. O. Box 713
Shelton, CT 06484
One Kingston Drive
Ansonia, CT 06401
(203) 735-6415, FAX (203) 736-9102

Kenneth W. Kubofcik, President
Alt.: John Sandusky

Specialists in radiation and acoustical products including unreinforced loaded vinyl noise barriers, reinforced loaded vinyl noise barriers, foil faced pipe wraps, floor mats, and composites.
"Falconcloth", "Falconmat", "Falconcoustic SK".

H. L. BLACHFORD, INC.
1855 Stephenson Highway
Troy, MI 48007-0397
(313) 689-7800

Jack Nicholas, President
Alt: Joseph McCarty, Nat. Sales Mgr.
West: Tom Pellegrino, 463 N. Smith Ave.
    Corona, CA 91720
    (714) 734-3360, FAX (714) 734-9711

A full line of acoustical materials for the OEM market and transportation industry. Noise treatments are available as vibration damping, "Aquaplas DL, DS, & DF", sound absorption "Conaflex", and sound barriers including "Baryfol", "Baryskin", and "Baryform". Many products are form molded, such as automotive dash sound insulators.

DIGISONIX,
Div. of Nelson Industries, Inc.
1415 Hwy. 51 West, P.O. Box 200
Stoughton, WI 53589-0200
(608) 873-1500, FAX (608) 873-1520

Steve Wise, General Manager

A manufacturer of active attenuation systems. Called Digisonix Digital Sound Cancellation Systems, they generate inverse sound waves which cancel low frequency noise. The system has proven effective in quieting duct-borne noise in HVAC systems, industrial fans, vacuum pumps and compressors. Other divisions of Nelson Industries, including Universal Silencer Division, manufacture exhaust and filtration systems for mobile equipment powered by gas or diesel engines, turbines, blowers and railroad locomotive engines.

ECKEL INDUSTRIES, INC.
Acoustical Division
155 Fawcett Street
Cambridge, MA 02138
(617) 491-3221, FAX (617) 547-2171

John W. Flood, Vice President
Alt. Alan Eckel, President

A manufacturer of noise control systems for machinery enclosures, barriers, and room sound absorption; acoustic materials and products for dampening and reducing equipment noise; hearing conservation and acoustic research rooms for audiological testing and chambers for product development and research. Trade names are; "Eckoustic", "TEC", "An-Eck-Oic Chambers".

G.F.C. FOAM CORPORATION
7401 South 78th Avenue
Bridgeview, IL 60455
(312) 496-8600/8601, FAX (708) 496-0028

Richard Lotesta,
Western Regional Sales Manager
Alt. John Chaya (714) 455-4931

A manufacturer of open-cell sound-absorptive polyurethane foam materials. Sales are primarily to fabricators who service OEM markets.

GENERAL FOAM OF MINNESOTA, INC.
1800 Como Ave.
St. Paul, MN 55108
(612) 645-0274, FAX (612) 645-7150

Niel Pedrolie
Joseph Pedrolie

A manufacturer of flexible polyurethane foam slab stock. The product line is made up of six types of polyester foam, and over thirty grades of polyether foam. The company also provides a complete line of foams flame bonded to vinyl, fabric, mylar and other substrates tailored to individual customer requirements. General Foam supplies converters with slab stock and rolls throughout the United States and Canada.

GREENWOOD FOREST PRODUCTS, INC. Darryl E. Jasmer, Sales Mgr.
5895 Southwest Jean Road
Lake Oswego, OR 97035
(503) 635-9271 or (800) 333-3898, FAX (503) 635-5399

A manufacturer of damped plywood called "dB-Ply". The dB-Ply panel can be worked with normal equipment and tools for applications such as flooring in multi-family construction, buses and railroad cars, and for floor, bulkheads, and decks in boat building.

ILLBRUCK
Sonex Acoustical Division
5155 E. River Rd. N.E., Suite 413
Minneapolis, MN 55421
(612) 521-3555, FAX (612) 572-1492

Larrie Reese, President
3800 Washington Ave.N.
Minneapolis, MN 55412
(612) 521-3555

A manufacturer of "Sonex", a porous acoustic melamine material that is an excellent sound absorber and meets class 1 regulations for flammability for a multitude of industrial acoustical applications. In concert with Architectural Surfaces, Inc., "Sonex" ceilings are available in a number of coatings and patterns.

PERSTORP COMPONENTS,
antiphon, inc.
2655 Woodward Ave.
Bloomfield Hills, MI 48013
(313) 332-0267 or (800) 431-8455, FAX (313) 332-0106

Peter Jackson,
Director of Technical Services
Alt. Richard Lynch, Vice Pres.
Alt. Dennis Huckins, Sales Mgr.

A manufacturer of "antiphon" and "Lay-Tech" noise control products including Absorbers, Dampers, and Barriers. "Antiphon SA" is a lightweight, fireproof sound absorber that will not burn or deteriorate. Antiphon LDA and LA are polyurethane foams. "Antiphon MPM, 13,D1D and LI-1-1/2B" are dampers composed of viscoelastic materials. They may be used with sheet steel, metals and wood as constrained layers or in combination with other materials. "Antiphon L-1/4" B, LB, LB-1 are barriers of loaded plastic sheets with various facings.

PRE FINISH METALS, INC.
Polycore Division
2111 E. Pratt Blvd.
Elk Grove Village, IL 60007
(312) 439-2210, FAX (708) 364-1008

Ed Vydra, PhD, Director R&D
Alt. Jim Shogren, Dir. Sales

A manufacturer of sound and vibration damping metal composites consisting of metal outer skins surrounding viscoelastic of film core material. Dissimilar metal skins can be used in composites up to .1250" thick, 50" wide. All materials produced in cost efficient continuous coil. Trade name is Polycore Composites.

THE SOUNDCOAT COMPANY
1 Burt Drive
Deer Park, NY 11729-5701
(516) 242-2246, FAX (516) 242-2246
        or
3002 Croddy Way
Santa Ana, CA 92799-5990
(714) 979-9202 FAX (714) 979-0834

Carl Wolaver, Market Manager
Alt: Francis Kirschner, Pres.

A manufacturer of acoustical materials including absorption, barrier, damping, gasketing and composites. Trade names for absorbers include: "Soundfoam" Embossed, Tedlar, Perforated Vinyl, "M," "Cabfoam" and Matte Film Finish. Barriers are "Soundmat FVP" and "Soundfab". Damping products are "Soundfoil Sheet Embossed," "Soundmat PB, M & LE," Embossed, and "Soundmat LFM." Gasketing is "Soundfoam CSB."

POLYMER TECHNOLOGIES, INC. Robert Prybutok, President
7006 Pencader Drive
Newark, DE 19702
(302) 738-9001, FAX (302) 738-9085

A manufacturer of noise absorbers, barriers and vibration dampers under the trademark "Polydamp." Absorbers include "Polydamp" Acoustical Foam (PAF) and Embossed Foam (PEF) a polyurethane foam core with optional film facings, pressure sensitive adhesives, and embossed surfaces. "Polydamp" Acoustical Barriers (PAB) are composed of a loaded vinyl barrier, a foam decoupling layer, and an optional pressure-sensitive adhesive backing with a variety of optional surfaces. Vibration dampers include "Polydamp" Extensional Damping Pad (EDP), Foil Dampers (PFD) composites of aluminum bonded to a viscoelastic adhesive backing and Noiseless Metal (PNM) composed of two layers of metal separated by a thin, viscoelastic polymer.

ASSOCIATE MEMBERS

ANATROL, INC. Ahid Nashif, President
10895 Indeco Drive
Cincinnati, OH 45241
(513) 793-8844, FAX (513) 793-0075

A noise and vibration consulting firm.

RIVERBANK ACOUSTICAL LABORATORIES Peter Straus, Engineer
Div. of IIT Research Institute Alt.: John Kopec, Supervisor
1512 Batavia
Geneva, IL 60134 (312) 232-0104

Riverbank is a recognized independent, accredited laboratory providing acoustical testing services including sound absorption, sound transmission loss, impact sound transmission, sound power, sound pressure levels, open plan/open offices, light reflectance, air flow resistance, impedance tube absorption, noise reduction of sound-isolating enclosures, and insertion loss measurements. Riverbank is frequently identified as the source of acceptable acoustical data in various commercial, civic, and military specifications. The laboratory houses a museum of acoustical memorabilia including an acoustical levitation device.

COMMITTEES

AWARDS
Chairman . . . . Ken Kubofcik
Member . . . . Richard Lotesta

NOISE CONTROL MANUAL
Chairman . . . . Bob Prybutok
Members. . . . . C. Wolovere, P. Jackson, L. Reese, D. Harris

EDUCATION
Chairman . . . . Ken Kubofcik
Members. . . . . Al Perez - Ilbruck, Dave Harris

FINANCE
Chairman . . . . Ken Kubofcik
Members . . . . Carl Wolovere, Dave Harris

LIAISON
Chairman . . . . Jack Nicholas
ASTM E-33, NCAC, ASA . . . Dave Harris
SAE . . . . Peter Jackson

LABELING IMPLEMENTATION (Inactive)

MEMBERSHIP DEVELOPMENT
Chairman . . . . John Flood
Members. . . . . All NCA Members

NOMINATING
Chairman . . . . Richard Lotesta
Member . . . . Rich Lynch

TECHNICAL
Chairman . . . . Peter Jackson
Members . . . . Peter Strauss, Dave Harris

Chapter 1 - NOISE CONTROL TECHNOLOGY

WHAT IS NOISE?

Noise is often defined as unwanted sound. It may be sound produced by an aircraft, punch press, stereo system, etc. In short, what is pleasing sound to one individual may be disturbing noise to another. To characterize sound, two parameters are generally required: sound pressure level and frequency. Examples of primary sound sources are vibrating surfaces and turbulent air (Figure 1-1).

Sound pressure level is a logarithmic quantity expressed in decibels (dB). It is related to the intensity or loudness of the sound (Table 1-1).

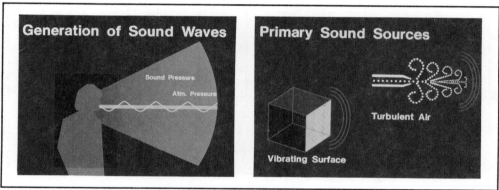

Figure 1-1. Sound Generation

Table 1-1 TYPICAL SOUND LEVELS

Sound source or environment	Decibels (dB)	Listener's perception
Jet aircraft at take-off	120	Threshold of pain
Boiler factory	110	Deafening
Noisy factory, loud street	90	Very loud
Noisy office, average factory	70	Loud
Average office, noisy home	50	Moderate
Private office, quiet conversation	30	Faint
Whisper	10	Very Faint

2 NOISE CONTROL MANUAL

Frequency describes the tonal quality of the sound or pitch and is expressed in units of cycles per second or Hertz (Hz). Often the range of hearing (50 to 15000 Hz) is broken into segments called octave bands. As such, the spectral character of sound can be graphically presented (Figure 1-2).

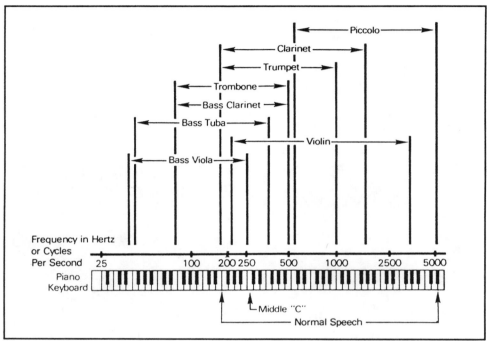

Figure 1-2 - Sound Frequency

See Appendix 1 for a complete set of definitions for acoustical and related terms.

MEASUREMENT OF SOUND

The basic measurement instrument in acoustics and noise control is the *sound level meter*. (Figure 1-3). With a hand held sound level meter, the overall sound level is measured in accordance with preselected weighing networks, i.e. A, B, & C. The C scale provides rather flat response from 50 to 5000 Hz, and the A and B scales sharply reduce the incident sound in the frequency range below 1000 Hz. (Figure 1-2). The A and B scales follow closely the response characteristics of the human ear and also the rate at which noise-induced hearing loss occurs. As such, all regulatory measurements involving health and safety (OSHA) or the acoustical environment (EPA) are obtained in the A scale mode of operation.

To obtain the octave band spectral character of the noise, an octave band analyzer, generally portable, or other more sophisticated instruments are utilized. In all cases, the measurements are given directly in decibels, i.e. db_A, dB_B, or dB_C, indicating the weighing scale utilized. It should be noted that for C scale measurements, the letter C is deleted by convention, that is, dB_C is expressed as dB.

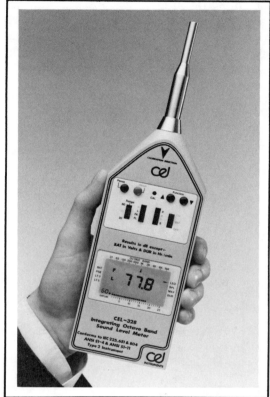

Figure 1-3 - Sound Level Meter

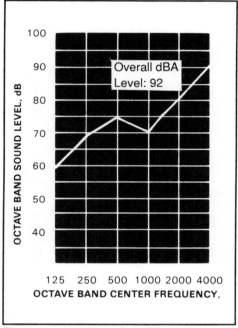

Figure 1-4 - Sound level varies with frequency

NOISE EXPOSURE LEVELS

Allowable noise exposure levels vary widely depending on the receiver situation. If you are trying to sleep in a very quiet country environment, a dripping faucet or cricket could be intolerable. In an office, if you know that you are being overheard or that you are intrusive to your neighbor will be unacceptable. The foregoing examples are not typically governed by regulations, albeit they are significant reason to implement noise control measures. In the United States of America and in most other industrialized nations, the Occupational Safety and Health Agency (OSHA) and the Environmental Protection Agency (EPA) have set limits on allowable noise exposure levels. Based on considerable study, these limits are generally indicative of the levels at which hearing loss will likely occur, or at which the noise will mask warning shouts. Primarily these are safety limits; annoyance limits are substantially lower.

4   NOISE CONTROL MANUAL

OSHA establishes the periods of time to which an individual may be exposed to different levels in excess of 90 dB$_A$ (Table 1-2). If a worker is exposed to several different noise levels during an 8-hour work day, the accumulative exposure for the day must be calculated or measured by a dosimeter (i.e. a cumulative measure of noise levels over time). Note that the OSHA limit is in effect 85 dB$_A$ since the law requires all workers exposed to 85 dB$_A$ for 8 hours to have audiometric testing on a yearly basis.

TABLE 1-2 ALLOWABLE OSHA NOISE EXPOSURE LEVELS

Noise Level, dB$_A$	Allowable daily exposure
85	8 hours
	audiometric testing of worker required
90	8 hours
92	6 hours
95	4 hours
97	3 hours
100	2 hours
102	1.5 hours
105	1 hour
110	0.5 hour
120	1 minute or less

TABLE 1-3 SUBJECTIVE PERCEPTION OF ACTUAL SOUND ENERGY CHANGE

Sound Pressure Level change	Subjective perception	Sound energy change
0 - 3 dB	Barely perceivable	50%
4 - 5 dB	Perceivable and significant	69%
6 dB	Resultant sound 1/4 lower than initial level	75%
7 - 9 dB	Major perceived reduction	87%
10 dB	Resultant sound 1/2 lower than initial level	90%

Noise exposures that exceed the criteria established by OSHA must be reduced below these limits to be in compliance. The methodology for reducing the noise may be "Engineering Controls" or "Management Controls". "Temporary Measures" such as personal ear protectors may be employed under certain circumstances for *limited periods* until engineering or management controls are implemented or in cases where there are no other practical methods. Engineering controls are the most common technique. The balance of this manual is, in essence, a study of the various ways one may implement engineering controls to meet the noise limits. Management controls, whereby the employee may have his work schedule structured so that the total time of the noise dose does not exceed the OSHA criteria, are a useful technique, however, most managers are unwilling to implement them since they upset normal work flow and reduce full utilization of experienced individuals.

Proper design of effective "engineering controls" cannot be achieved from A scale sound level meter readings alone. One must know the frequency content as well as the sound level of the offending noise to ensure satisfactory performance of noise control measures. Therefore, in addition to taking A scale sound level meter readings, octave band noise level measurements should also be made (Figure 1-4). An octave or one-third (1/3) band filter, used in conjunction with a sound level meter, measures the noise level of a group of frequencies. These levels provide a better indication of the nature of the noise and will enable the designer of the noise control measures to be more efficient in selecting the most economical solution. For example, if the noise is concentrated in one frequency band, noise control measures that are most effective for that band may be utilized. Without this information, broad band measures may be required at considerable extra expense.

> **OSHA COMPLIANCE REQUIREMENTS**
>
> - **ENGINEERING CONTROLS**
>
>   lower noise level to 85 dB$_A$
>
> - **MANAGEMENT CONTROLS**
>
>   limit worker time (Table 1-2)
>
> - **TEMPORARY MEASURES**
>
>   use ear protectors until permanent measures are implemented. (60 days)

BASIC PRINCIPLES OF NOISE CONTROL

There are three basic elements to be considered in controlling noise:

- Controlling or attenuating noise at its *source*;
- Controlling or attenuating noise along its *path* from source to listener;
- Controlling or attenuating noise at the *receiver* (listener).

Thus, in industrial noise control, reference is made to SPR (Source, Path, Receiver) control. Any noise control problem may require that one, two or all three of these basic control elements be taken into consideration.

There are three primary ways to control noise:

- The noise source can be selected, redesigned or modified to operate more quietly, and/or resiliently supported to prevent the transmission of vibration.

- Sound energy can be absorbed by a porous acoustical material, or blocked along its path.

- Sound energy can be confined to, or excluded from, an enclosure.

Control of the source is most easily handled by purchasing quiet equipment. Original equipment manufacturers (OEM) can, with sometimes minimal cost, implement substantial noise control measures in the design stage. Even add-on noise control elements are usually more effective in terms of "decibels per dollar" (dB/$) than post-control efforts. Well-balanced and smooth running machinery is usually quieter and will have a longer life. Both active and passive noise suppressors (i.e. mufflers) are available or easily adapted to many engines, etc. Noisy equipment can also be quieted on installation with the proper use of noise isolating pads, mounts or damping materials.

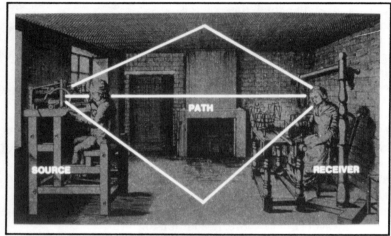

Figure 1-5 Source, Path and Receiver

SOURCE CONTROL = Most Effective dB/$

Absorbing sound along the path can be effective when the room has very hard surface materials. Painted concrete, wallboard, stucco and masonry are very sound-reflective materials. When used extensively in a space, sound will tend to reverberate or bounce causing amplification of noise sources. The addition of soft porous materials that are efficient sound absorbers will reduce the "reverberation time" or echoes. The result will be a much more acoustically desirable space. However, the overall reduction of the noise source usually will not exceed 10-12 decibels.

Most acoustical materials absorb sound by converting acoustical energy to heat due to air friction in the cells or passages of the materials. Soft fibrous or flexible foam materials are typically good sound absorbers. Other sound absorbing principals are discussed in the sound absorbing materials section.

When the path is a duct, efficient sound absorbing materials will reduce the signal each time it bounces. As sound is transmitted down the duct, a sound absorbing lining attenuates the

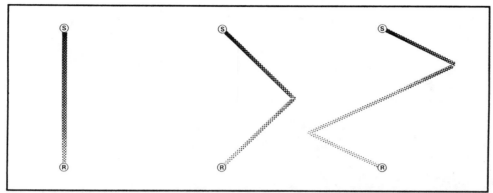

Figure 1-6 - Direct, single and multiple reflection paths from source to receiver.

sound by absorbing it along the perimeter walls. The more effective the absorber, the more sound attenuation will be achieved.

To be effective in confining noise within an enclosure, or in excluding it, the walls, ceilings and floors of such an enclosure should have high sound transmission loss values. Sound transmission loss is best expressed in dB at one-third or octave band center frequencies. Adding sound absorbing materials to the interior of an enclosure will improve overall noise reduction.

Regarding effective sound barrier materials, original thinking was to make it as heavy and limp as possible. Considerable research on composite materials and systems of construction have shown that other physical properties improve the sound barrier characteristics well beyond the "mass law" principals (i.e. for every doubling of the mass there is a 5 dB improvement in transmission loss). A key to success with high performance transmission loss materials and systems is to assure that no sound leaks or flanking paths exist at joints, corners or acoustically weak spots. Partial height barriers or those that do not extend from wall to wall will never attenuate more sound than will diffract around the ends/edges.

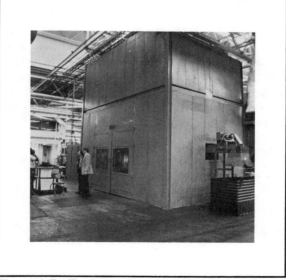

Figure 1-7 - Enclosure/barriers should be a heavy limp mass with an absorber on the source side.

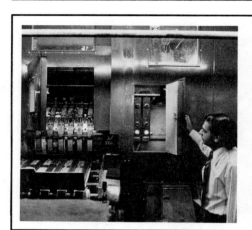 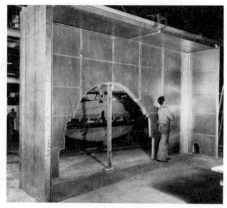

Figure 1-8 - Barriers must have no sound leaks or flanking paths.

SUMMARY

Noise is unwanted sound. Noise can be controlled by addressing the source, path and/or receiver. Measures that reduce the noise level at the source are the most effective in terms of decibels reduction per dollar invested (dB/$). Source control measures include well balanced, smooth operating equipment, damping, resilient mounts, mufflers and enclosures. Receiver controls are the second most effective noise control measures and include enclosures for the receiver, and temporary measures such as ear attenuators or ear plugs. Only when all the practical means of source and receiver controls have been implemented should path controls be implemented. Mitigation of noise along the path includes applying sound absorption materials on surfaces that could reflect sounds and constructing noise barriers such as walls, floor/ceiling systems, etc. Engineering controls that reduce noise levels below 85 dB_A are required by OSHA regulations.

****

Chapter 2 - SOUND ABSORBING MATERIALS

MATERIAL TYPES

Materials for noise and vibration control may be broadly classified into those applicable for treatment of the source, for reduction along the noise path and for receiver treatment. Since one is concerned with a dynamic energy source, a multitude of paths, and a human receiver that is highly mobile and sensitive, material types are innumerable. Complicating matters further, some materials are used extensively at all three locations in the noise equation, namely the source, path and receiver. For this reason we have chosen to categorize material types as follows:

- Absorbing Materials - those that dissipate or convert sound energy on impact.

- Barrier Materials - those that block sound waves.

- Vibration isolation/damping materials - those that reduce radiated sound.

- Silencers, passive and active - those that suppress sounds.

A change in process or redesign of equipment is generally conducted by the manufacturer who may elect to utilize any one or all of these categories to reduce noise emissions. Noise path treatment is often the only practical means available to a noise control engineer. Depending on the specific circumstances, any or all of the material types may be effective. However, most solutions utilize absorbing and barrier materials. Noise control efforts at the receiver may utilize any or all the materials.

Sound absorptive materials typically have a soft, porous structure, offer only low resistance to a sound wave, and permit the passage of the sound to the other side relatively un-attenuated. Effective sound absorbers of fibrous base materials generally convert sound energy into minute quantities of heat that are easily dissipated. However there are several other physical phenomena that will substantially reduce reflected sound energy. Other materials and principles include diaphragm absorbers and Helmholtz resonators. An important consideration of all efficient sound absorbers is that they are poor sound barriers. Early acoustician's evaluated absorbers by measuring the rate that air passed through the material. In fact, some sound absorbing materials are still classified by their resistance to air passage in "rayles". Since some materials are both good absorbers and resist air passage, a better rating system evolved. We now measure the sound absorption coefficients of a material and classify them by the Noise Reduction Coefficient (NRC). See the appendix for a more detailed explanation of NRC.

By contrast, typical sound barrier materials are hard, heavy and very reflective. They resist the passage of sound through them and they are poor sound absorbers. Lead is a well known example of a good sound barrier. Barrier materials generally follow what is referred to as the mass law. For each doubling of the mass theoretical predictions indicate an increase of 5 dB in the sound reduction or sound transmission loss. Since mass is a costly way to achieve good sound transmission loss, new materials and systems have been developed. The best acoustical barriers in present day technology utilize a combination of materials formed into a composite or system.

A vibration damping material reduces the vibration intensity of a sound source so that it does not radiate noise. A good example of damping is the effect of placing your hand on a vibrating sheet metal panel of a mechanical device such as a dishwasher. Your hand is soft, pliable and adds mass. If placed at the correct location, significant reductions in noise can be obtained.

A vibration isolation material prevents the vibration of one object from being transferred to another object. The two objects are isolated from one another using springs or resilient mounts. Since sound originates when some form of energy sets up oscillations in air or other media, it is clear that if either the vibrating energy or the number of vibrating objects is reduced, the sound will be reduced.

Silencers are of two types: passive and active. Passive silencers include the common auto mufflers and many unique add on devices to suppress specific noise sources. Active silencers are a new and exciting noise control technology. By creating sound waves that are out of phase with the original noise, wave theory indicates the sound will be canceled. The concept has become practical only with the advent of sophisticated and now relatively inexpensive computers.

SOUND ABSORPTIVE MATERIALS

To be an efficient sound absorber, a material usually will convert impinging acoustic energy to some other form of energy, usually heat. There are three major types of absorbers; porous absorptive materials, diaphragmatic absorbers, and resonant or reactive absorbers.

<u>Porous absorptive materials</u> are the best known of the acoustical absorbers. They are usually fuzzy, fibrous materials, foams, fabrics, carpets, cushions, etc. Cork was the first material utilized commercially for sound absorption in architectural applications. Soon after, bagasse, a sugar cane byproduct was formed into tiles with a binder. Later, wood fiber tiles and boards appeared. Today, most of the commercial materials are a mineral or glass fiber board made on wet and dry process forming equipment. These materials are available in light density blankets, boards and composites (Figure 2-1). Open cell foams, utilizing foamed polyurethane, isocyranurate, and ceramic fibers were recently introduced as sound absorbers. In all of these materials, absorption occurs by causing the sound waves to activate motion of the fibers, membranes and the air in the spaces surrounding the fibers or voids. Frictional

energy losses generate heat, which is dissipated, thereby reducing the acoustic energy. Some scattering also occurs within the materials adding to the reduction of acoustic energy (Figure 2-2).

Material properties that affect sound absorption efficiency, in order of importance are: thickness, density, porosity or flow resistance, coefficient of elasticity, and acoustic impedance. In all materials, thickness is the most important aspect.

In <u>glass fiber absorbers</u>, having a range of 1 to 8 lb. density, increasing thickness is 10 times more efficient in improving absorption characteristics than altering any other physical property. For the same thickness glass fiber products, smaller glass fiber diameter size will improve absorption in many frequency bands. AA size fibers are typically used in aircraft where weight and thickness are limited. Increasing density will improve sound absorption is some frequency bands. Resin content will change the stiffness of the fibers

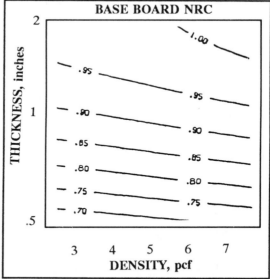

Figure 2-1 - Fiberglass blankets, boards and composites.

causing positive and negative effects depending on the frequency. Flow resistance of the base material has some effect but is overshadowed by the foregoing(Figure 2-3).

In <u>foam materials</u>, thickness will also dramatically affect the sound absorption characteristic. Note that only open cell foams are efficient sound absorbers. Rigid foams, used primarily for thermal insulation, generally have considerable flow resistance and thereby block the sound from entering the material. Density will affect the absorption

Figure 2-2 - Sound absorption of fiberglass materials.

characteristics at certain frequencies since density affects cell size and membrane thickness (Figure 2-4).

Note that *facing materials will tend to block sound* from entering all foam and fibrous materials and significantly reduce the potential for absorption in many frequencies. Generally, facings greater than 1 mill thickness with a high flow resistance will be detrimental. Open weave

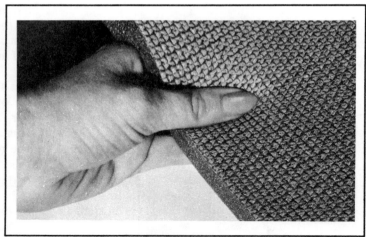

Figure 2-3 - Open cell foam absorbers

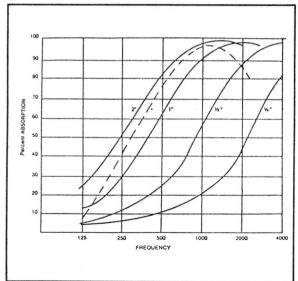

Figure 2-4 - Open cell foam absorption

cloth materials and facings with a 20% or greater open area tend to maintain (not adversely affect) the sound absorption characteristics for most fibrous and foam sound absorbers at normal frequencies. With careful design, some thin facings may even enhance sound absorption at certain frequencies since they now function as a diaphragm.

Diaphragm Absorbers: In a diaphragmatic absorber, the panel oscillates at the frequencies in the impinging sound wave. If the sound waves coincide with the natural frequencies of the particular absorber the panel will be in a resonant condition and therefore have a relatively large vibration amplitude. This vibration will cause the panel to dissipate some of its energy through damping and radiation. The panel therefore acts as an absorber having maximum absorption characteristics at its fundamental frequency (and higher harmonics) which depend upon the geometry of the panel and its damping characteristics. In sheet materials, this effect takes place at low frequencies, usually in the range of 40 to 300 Hz. However, placing a thin membrane against a perforated sheet will yield the same effect at other frequencies. This approach to sound absorption can provide efficient absorption at specific frequencies.

If a panel is hung in front of a hard wall at a small distance from the wall, the air space will act as a compliant element (spring) giving rise to a resonant system comprised of the panel's lumped mass and the air compliance.

The absorption performance of such a panel absorber can be enhanced both in absorption magnitude and effective frequency range by installing a porous sound absorptive material, such as open cell foam or fibrous glass in the air space between the panel and the wall.

Typical panel absorbers include gypsum board partitions, wood paneling, windows, suspended ceilings, ceiling reflectors, and stretched membranes over a perforated stiff panel. However, since the absorption coefficient of this absorber type is very dependent on mass, rigidity, size, shape, and mounting methods, it is difficult to forecast how any particular panel will operate in practice. Usually it is necessary to test prototypes for each specific application.

Resonant Absorbers: Resonant or reactive absorbers (often called Helmholtz resonators) are cavities which confine a volume of air which is connected to the atmosphere by a small hole or channel in the cavity. If the cavity is very small compared with the wave length of the incident sound wave, the air in the connecting channel is forced to oscillate into and out of the cavity. This type of absorber has a very narrow frequency band where absorption takes place, thereby limiting its use.

Generally, practicality limits the size of a Helmholtz resonator so they are mostly used for frequencies below 400 Hz. Their sharp resonance-type absorption makes them useful when very selective absorption is required, such as a break squeal noise. If tolerable, some reduced absorption at the resonance frequency can be considerably broadened by adding a resonance damping material such as foam or glass fiber into the neck or into the cavity.

Perforated Panel Absorbers: Perforated panel absorbers can be thought of as a large number of individual Helmholtz resonators. When a perforated panel is spaced away from a solid backing, the holes in the panel constitute the necks of the individual resonators, which share the common volume behind the panel as their cavities. Also, just as with a single Helmholtz resonator, a porous air space behind the panel will add damping to the system. This damping will reduce the amount of absorption at the resonance peak but will broaden the frequency range over which the panel will be an effective sound absorber.

Because the perforations become acoustically transparent at low frequencies due to diffraction, the sound absorption properties of the porous blanket are only slightly affected in the lower frequency range. However, the panel solid areas will reflect the shorter wavelength sounds such that the higher frequency range sound absorption can be severely reduced.

For broadening the frequency range over which useful absorption can be achieved, the panel can be perforated with holes of differing sizes and/or the panel can be mounted at an angle to the backing plate.

Spray-on Absorbers: Spray-on absorbers consist of a range of materials formed from mineral or synthetic organic fibers mixed with a binding agent to hold the fibrous material together. (Note: Early versions of these materials contained asbestos. Do not utilize any form containing asbestos as it has been declared a health hazard. Check with the manufacturer before using.) Most common are rock wool, glass fiber, perlite, paper pulp and an array of similar porous, lightweight volcanic granules or fibers. During spraying, the material is mixed with a binding agent and water to produce a soft lightweight material with a coarse surface texture and high sound absorbing characteristics. This material may be applied directly to a wide number of surfaces including wood, concrete, metal lath, steel, and galvanized metal. Some are used for fireproofing in commercial buildings.

When sprayed onto a solid backing, the materials exhibit good mid and high frequency absorption and when applied to metal lath with an air space behind it, the material also exhibits good low frequency absorption. Spray-on depths of up to two (2) inches are common. Absorption characteristics vary widely depending on density, porosity, and face sealing. In some instances, the sprayed surface is over-punched with a multitude of small holes to improve the ability of the sound to penetrate into the material and/or increase surface area.

Care must be exercised when applying spray-on absorbers since the absorption characteristics are dependent upon the amount and type of binding agent used and the way it is mixed during the spray-on process. If too much binder is used, the material becomes too hard, or a surface skin develops, resulting in poor sound absorption. If too little binder is employed, the material will be prone to disintegration. With less material and a low flow resistance, it will also not be a good absorber. Most spray-on materials possess good fire resistance and thermal resistance properties. However, some pulp base materials have been known to "punk" causing concern for use in incombustible buildings. Spray-on materials tend to seal joints and cracks thereby improving the sound transmission characteristics of a building system. Do not expect high performance, however, since these materials are not good sound barriers themselves.

Spray-on materials have been successfully used for broadband sound absorption in a variety of architectural spaces including schools, gymnasiums, auditoriums, and in a variety of industrial applications such as machine shops and power plants. Durability, cleanability and uniformity are clearly limited. For this reason, these materials are painted. Paint films will significantly reduce their sound absorption properties. A "non-bridging" spray paint, when applied in a fashion that will not impede penetration of the sound, can be used successfully. However, the resultant application will not always retain the initial sound absorption properties. Spray on materials will also have poor aesthetics and poor durability.

Absorption Material/Product Specifications

Most of the foregoing materials and applications are specified by pertinent industry standards. A list of related ASTM Standards is in Appendix 2.

Sound Absorption Testing

Most sound absorption testing is done in a laboratory using the "Reverberation Room." The random incidence absorption coefficients are determined at a specific frequency band by measuring the rate of decay of a sound in a highly reverberant room. The test procedure is specified and described in ASTM Standard C-423, "Standard Test Method for Sound Absorption and Sound Absorption Coefficients by the Reverberation Room Method." (Figure 2-5)

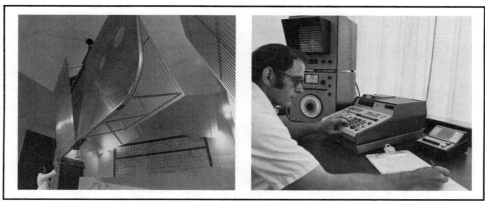

Figure 2-5 - Sound absorption test in Reverberation Room

The reverberation chamber is a large masonry cube with a preferred volume of 7063 cubic feet. Designs are intended to create a "diffuse" sound field so that generated sound waves theoretically impinge on the specimen at all angles of incidence during the steady state and decaying sound signal. Diffusion is achieved by means of turning vanes, special panels and non-parallel walls. Interior surfaces are highly sound reflective and the chamber is constructed to be isolated from intruding noise. A test specimen consisting of 72 square feet is constructed on mountings that simulate various typical applications. Note that the mounting will significantly affect sound absorption performance. For example, a ceiling board placed flat on the floor will not have the effect of the 16" air cavity behind the same ceiling material in an E-405 mounting (Figure 2-6 and performance data in Appendix 4).

The total absorption in the room is first measured without the specimen by turning on a sound source long enough for the sound level to come to a steady state. The source is suddenly turned off and the time required for the sound to decay to a set level is recorded. Called the reverberation time, a long decay rate indicates little absorption is present. After measuring the empty room, the specimen is placed in the room and a similar measurement is conducted. The absorption added to the room by the test specimen is then determined by taking the difference. Absorption coefficients are measured at specified frequency bands by dividing the total absorption by the area of the specimen ($\alpha = A/S$ where α (alpha) is the absorption coefficient, A is the total absorption and S is the area of the specimen).

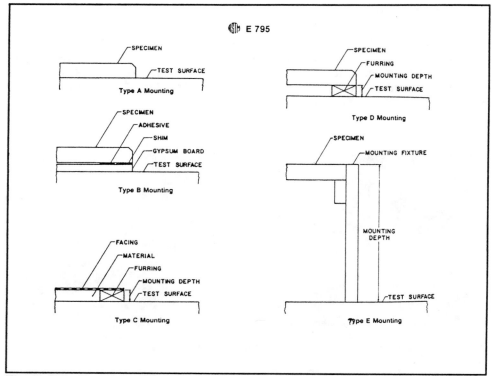

Figure 2-6 - Examples of ASTM E795 mountings for sound absorption tests.

The frequency dependence of the absorption coefficient is obtained by measuring the absorption in six one-third octave bands centered at 125, 250, 500, 1000, 2000 and 4000 Hz. The laboratory report will therefore show six absorption coefficients and the frequency at which they were measured. These numbers are rounded to the nearest integral multiple of 0.01. While vital to most determinations of room absorption, it is somewhat cumbersome to compare absorbers if one must be looking at six numbers for each of them. To simplify such comparisons and to provide a means of rating the sound absorbing properties of a material, a one-number rating scheme is employed called the Noise Reduction Coefficient (NRC). NRC is calculated by averaging the absorption coefficients at the four measuring frequencies of 250, 500, 1000 and 2000 Hz. (those in the speech range).

A convenient way to describe sound absorption coefficients is to call them "percent sound absorption". While an excellent descriptor, it is in fact not precise. Note that both the sound absorption coefficients and the NRC are reported as a decimal starting at 0 and extending to something slightly in excess of 1. As more efficient materials were developed it was determined that values greater than 1 (or 100 %) are readily obtainable. Early data rounded all numbers in excess of 1.00 to 1.00. Present test criteria require that actual measurements

Sound Absorbing Materials 17

be reported. Consequently, some efficient absorption materials have both sound absorption coefficients and NRC's greater than 1.00. These numbers are correctly used in making room calculations (Appendix 3).

Specimen mountings can significantly affect the sound absorption coefficients and the NRC. For this reason it is imperative to identify the mounting method or designation (Figure 2-6) when providing test data or comparing materials. For example, a 1" thick 3# density glass fiber board will achieve an NRC .70 when tested on a "Type A" mounting (i.e. directly against a solid backing) while this same material when tested on an "E-405" mounting (i.e. with a 16" air space behind the material) has an NRC .75. The sound absorption coefficients at 125 Hz. are .11 for the type A mounting and .32 for the E-405 mounting. Other materials may vary even more. Mountings are specified for ceiling systems, wall panels, space absorbers, office screens, drapes, and nearly every normal situation. While there is some uniformity between the NRCs for the various mountings, these values should only be used for general comparisons. *Caution: specifications should identify the mounting.*

Other tests for sound absorption have been adopted. However, ASTM C-423 is universal in the industry. The impedance tube, ASTM Designation C-384, Standard Test method for Impedance and Absorption of Acoustical Materials by the Impedance Tube Method is useful for initial screening of materials. There is no established correlation between C-384 and C-423 (Appendix 2).

Laboratory reports should be carefully scrutinized when selecting materials for their sound absorption characteristics. To be in compliance with ASTM C-423 test procedures the test report must provide:

- a complete description of the product and identify all attributes that may affect acoustical performance (i.e. manufacturer's identification by product name or number is insufficient)
- sound absorption coefficients at the six center frequencies from 125 to 4000 Hz. plus the NRC
- the test procedure used with any deviations
- the mounting used in the test

To assure test compliance and reliable data, look for laboratories that have met the criteria established for the National Voluntary Laboratory Accreditation Program (NVLAP).

Sound absorption measurements at specific angle of incidence are made in a laboratory environment that is semi-anechoic, or nearly devoid of sound reflections. Acoustically, the semi-anechoic test room is diametrically opposed to the reverberation room. All surfaces except the test specimen are nearly perfect absorbers. Sound source signals are carefully selected to be directive and to simulate spreading patterns similar to human speech. No diffusers are used. Specimens are place in the "primary flanking position." In the case of a ceiling evaluation, an idealized screen of specific dimensions and sound barrier characteristics

18 NOISE CONTROL MANUAL

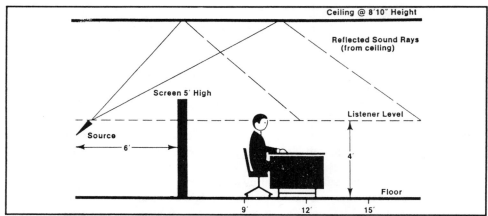

Figure 2-7 - Open office chamber tests sound absorption at specific angles

divides the test chamber. Only reflected sounds that bounce off the ceiling specimen centered over the divider are measured. A similar setup is configured for evaluating wall materials or office screens for sounds that may reflect from these surfaces into an adjacent work station. Sound attenuation data is acquired at specified frequencies typical of speech by subtracting the receiver level from the source level. Measurements of the source signal are taken in the immediate field of the specified sound signal. Receiver measurements are made along a specific path typical of the location a human receiver may occupy in an adjoining work station (Figure 2-7).

A more detailed description of the procedures is presented in Appendix 2. While designed for evaluating products and systems in the open plan office, these procedures are eminently useful for evaluating the flanking sound characteristics of materials in an industrial environment. A broader frequency band of sound sources typical of the industrial environment may be needed (i.e. 125 to 5000 Hz.).

SOME SPECIFIC ABSORPTION MATERIALS - Comments

The most common absorbing materials are glass or mineral fibers and plastic foam.

Foam materials with an open cell structure generally exhibit excellent sound absorption characteristics. They also can provide vibration isolation and damping. However, they are usually poor sound barriers unless they incorporate a barrier septum. Ester types of polyurethane foams are most commonly used for noise reduction. Flexible foams are available in reticulated open-pore construction or non-reticulated with a microporous integral skin left intact. The non-reticulated foam has extremely thin membranes closing off the spaces between the strains. Closed cell foams, usually considered rigid foams, are excellent for thermal insulation. However, closed cell foams generally have poor sound absorption characteristics.

Foams with convoluted surfaces and compressed felt-like foams are also manufactured to maximize absorption in specific frequency regions. Two (2) lb/ft^3 density foam is normally used for sound absorption. Flame retardant additives, protective films for dirty or oily environments, and high density flexible sound barriers are common options. Note that the protective films and barrier backings may have a significant effect on sound absorption.

Members of NCA manufacture and market a wide array of foam absorbers (Figure 2-8). To identify and choose the correct product for your application, you should contact the manufacturers directly. In general, foam materials are flexible, easily cut, are available in various colors and, depending on thickness and density, they provide a wide range of sound absorption. While specific products will vary, foams generally have limited temperature applications and may produce undesirable off-gassing under fire conditions. Many new and proprietary products have been developed to alleviate these limitations.

Glass fiber absorbing materials are composed of long fibers bonded together with resin or other bonding agents. Generally considered a dry manufacturing process, glass fibers are spun much like cotton candy and blown onto a conveyer. Resin is typically introduced on the fibers as they are blown. As the uncured fibers progress down the conveyer, they are compressed to the desired density, typically from 0.5 lb. to 6 lb., and proceed through an oven for curing. The light density materials are blankets while rigid boards are generally of heavier density. Some facings are applied in line. For heavier density glass fiber boards, from 12 to 40 lb., uncured wool is placed in heated platen presses to cure. Called molded board, the press platens may be fabricated to provide intricate shaped parts.

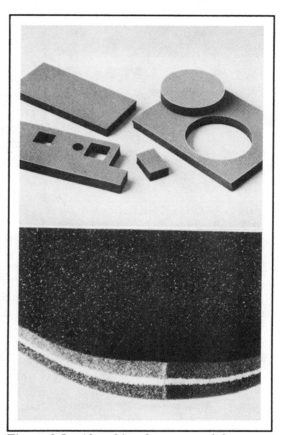

Figure 2-8 - Absorbing foam materials

Light density blanket glass fiber materials are widely used for building insulation. Medium density boards are generally used in commercial equipment, for ceiling boards, and in a wide range of building product applications. High-density materials are used for molded acoustical liners in vehicles and specialty equipment insulation. Since glass melts at approximately 1200

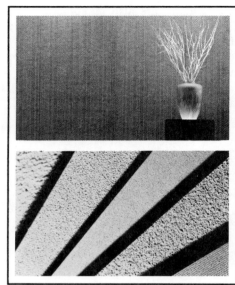

Figure 2-9 - Glass fiber base, cloth faced wall & ceiling boards.

degree F., glass fiber materials are usually considered incombustible and may be used in medium temperature applications. As more resin is introduced, both the fire ratings and temperature limits will be compromised.

The sound absorption characteristics of glass fiber materials, in the norm, are excellent. However, like foam, they are poor sound barriers. Increasing density may improve barrier characteristics but will also decrease absorption. Protective facings of open weave cloth and films are used for ceiling tile and wall panel applications. Some composites utilize glass fiber materials and high density barrier materials to provide dual attributes. Glass fiber boards and blankets are utilized to fabricate a wide range of finished acoustical products including ceiling and wall systems, space absorbers, wall fillers and anechoic chambers. NRCs of .70 are typical for 3/4" boards and 2" boards may exceed 1.00 (Figure 2-9).

Fine glass fiber materials have been used extensively in the aircraft industry. While more expensive, the finer (i.e. smaller in diameter) fibers have upgraded acoustical and thermal properties, making them acceptable for applications having significant weight and space restrictions (see Appendix 4 for test data on glass fiber materials).

Mineral fibers are used in two forms for acoustical applications. The most widely recognized is the formed mineral tile for ceiling board (Figure 2-10). Mineral blankets are also widely used as thermal and acoustical blankets. Mineral blankets are manufactured in much the same fashion as glass fiber materials. Molten rock wool is formed into fine fibers held together with a binder. The process is not conducive to making board products. Ceiling board basic is fabricated using rock wool fibers formed on a wet process line. The Fordrinier process uses a wet mix of mineral wool, water, and water soluble binders. This slurry is spread out on a moving screen where excess water is drained. Much like a paper mill, the 12 foot wide damp mass is then roll formed to thickness of 5/8" or 3/4" and dried in a series of ovens. These boards are then fabricated on equipment that places fissures, pin holes, cuts to size, fabricates special edge details, spray-paints faces, and packages the boards. Most product is nominal 2' x 2' or 4' lay-in ceiling board and 12" x 12" Tongue & Groove (T&G) ceiling tile.

Mineral ceiling boards have NRCs in the range of 0.45 to 0.65. With a density of nominally 15 lbs. the boards have decent sound barrier characteristics. These boards are also used in some composite materials applications. With a melting point of over 2000 degrees F, mineral fiber products have excellent fire resistant properties. They are widely used in commercial buildings. Mineral blankets are primarily used as acoustical insulation fillers in partition and floor/ceiling assembly voids for upgraded sound barrier performance (Figure 2-10).

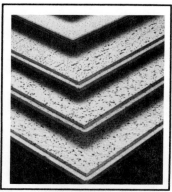

Figure 2-10 - Mineral ceiling tile

Other sound absorptive materials include cork, wood fiber boards, cellulose insulation and a whole range of high tech fibrous materials. Cork and wood fiber board are still used in residential units where flamespread ratings are not a deterrent. Used as sound absorbing ceiling and wall treatments these materials are the forerunner of the glass and mineral products described above. Wood fiber boards are made on a wet process machine. These boards are then fabricated into lay-in ceiling boards and tile with a wide range of patterns and finishes. Sound absorption properties are in the 0.45 to 0.55 NRC range. These materials only achieve their sound absorptive ratings when they are fissured, punched, or drilled to increase the surface area and allow sound to penetrate the fibers. Wood fiber boards, primarily designed as exterior sheathing, is also utilized as a "sound deadening board" in wall and floor/ceiling systems that separate living units.

Ceramic fibers and other related high tech materials have emerged as interesting sound absorptive alternatives in recent years. With relatively high price tags, these materials have superior resistance to high temperature environments such as those found in power plants. They are used extensively in mufflers and jet engine nacelles for both thermal and acoustical insulation.

Specialty absorbers that utilize the Helmholtz resonator and diaphragmatic absorbing principals are discussed in a previous section.

Chapter 3 - SOUND BARRIER MATERIALS/SYSTEMS

SOUND BARRIER FUNCTION

It is well-known that a wall or heavy enclosure can serve as a very effective barrier against airborne sound transmission. While any surface will reflect some of the sound which reaches it, only heavy, acoustically designed materials and systems with airtight surfaces are significantly effective in "stopping" sound. The effectiveness of a barrier depends on the

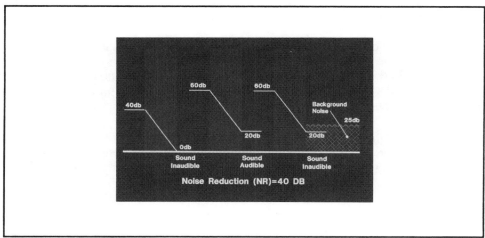

Figure 3-1 - Noise reduction via barrier

weight, stiffness, mounting, damping, the use of single or multiple panels, the spacing of these panels, and the use of absorptive material in the cavities.

The function of a sound barrier is to provide a means of maintaining a difference in sound level between spaces (Figure 3-1). If a higher level, say 60 dB, exists on one side of a wall, while an acceptable level on the opposite side is not more than 20 dB, the wall must provide at least 40 dB isolation or noise reduction (also called sound transmission loss) to keep out the intruding sound. If the wall provides 40 dB noise reduction, the intruding sound will be at a level of 20 dB or 5 dB below a receiving room ambient sound level of 25 dB. A barrier that reduces the sound source to a level that is lower than the existing ambient level in the receiving room will not be heard (e.g. The level is said to have a 0 signal to noise ratio if intruding sounds are masked by the background sounds. By contrast, source sounds that are well above the background noise are clearly heard and have a positive signal to noise ratio). Thus, a sound barrier, be it a wall, floor, or partition, should provide enough noise reduction or sound transmission loss to keep intruding sound below the desired level in the space that it is protecting.

When a sound wave strikes a barrier, the barrier is set into motion. The barrier then becomes a sound source and sets into motion the air on the other side. Some of the energy is reflected back toward the source, and some is lost in moving the partition.

Sound Transmission Loss

The ratio of the sound energy incident upon one surface of a partition to the energy radiated from the opposite surface is called the "sound transmission loss" of the partition. The actual energy "loss" is partially reflected energy (back toward the source) and partially heat (internal losses within the partition).

Sound transmission loss is an inherent characteristic of a barrier and is essentially independent of the location of the barrier. Since the barrier moves with an oscillating and accelerated motion, it obviously requires force to initiate and sustain the motion. The partition has mass; it is accelerated by the force or pressure of the impinging sound wave. Therefore, it is possible to analyze its motion mathematically.

If the barrier were a "limp" mass, and moved only back and forth (like the end of a piston), the sound transmission loss for energy randomly incident on the barrier (excluding losses at the edge of the panel and any "leaks") would be calculated as:

$$TL = 10\log_{10}[1 + \frac{\pi f m \cos\theta}{pc}]^2$$

where: TL = Transmission Loss (dB)
       f = Frequency (Hz)
       m = superficial mass of the partition (lbs.)
       p = density of air (#/cu. ft.)
       c = speed of sound in air (fps)
       π = 3.14
       θ = angle of incident sound (degrees)

This equation shows that the transmission loss of a barrier is dependent on the frequency of the sound, the angle of incidence of the sound wave, and mass of the barrier. Note that the Transmission Loss is greatest for sound incident normally on the surface (cos $0°$ = 1) and least for sound impinging on the surface at grazing incidence (cos $90°$ = 0). For most practical applications, the sound is incident over a large range of angles and this equation can be integrated over a range of angles for any given sound situation. Generally, however, one can assume a common range of angles of incidence (e.g. $0°$ - $78°$), in which case the expression for Transmission Loss reduces to:

TL = 20 log(fw) - 47.5 dB

where f is the frequency in Hz and w is the superficial weight of the barrier in kg/m^2. From this formula it is easy to recognize that for a doubling of either the frequency or the mass the Transmission Loss will increase 6 dB. This is the well known form of the "mass law." Unfortunately, few materials or systems of construction conform to mass law principles. Masonry and lead are about at the limit. Composite wall systems exhibit a complex sound transmission loss characteristic. A 2 by 4 wood stud wall with gypsum board faces has 2 "coincidence dips" and generally performs better than predicted by the mass law (Figure 3-2).

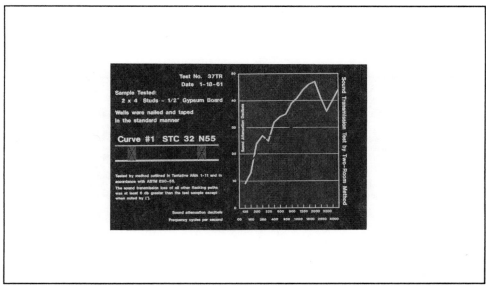

Figure 3-2 - Sound Transmission Loss(Class) for a conventional wall system.

Resonances - In addition to the coincidence resonance, a barrier panel possesses other resonant properties. Like any physical system the panel has mass and some elasticity, and therefore natural vibration nodes exist. The number of modes and the frequencies at which a panel resonates depend on its size, mass and stiffness, and on the method of fixing at the edges. Of these frequencies, the fundamental or lowest is usually the most important in practice and is commonly referred to simply as the resonance frequency.

In most cases the size and material of the partition are such that the resonance frequency is well below the lowest frequency of interest. However, the possibility of a smaller panel having a resonance frequency which is within the range of interest must be borne in mind.

Below the resonance frequency, the insulation of the partition is largely stiffness-controlled, i.e., it acts as a spring rather than as an inertial load to the incident sound wave, with the result being that the insulation increases as the frequency is reduced.

When the frequency of the incident sound wave corresponds to a resonant frequency of the partition, very little energy is required to force the panel to vibrate. The resulting high amplitude of vibration produces a correspondingly high sound pressure level on the opposite side of the panel. In some instances the sound wave seems to pass through the panel almost as if it were not there. To avoid the effects of resonance, it is desirable to have the lowest natural frequency possible. This condition is favored by using panels which are as limp and massive as possible. However, 4 ft. by 8 ft. sheets of gypsum board also have a first panel resonance well below the frequency range of interest for building acoustics.

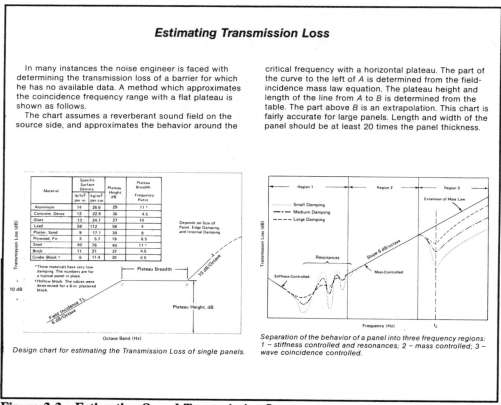

Figure 3-3 - Estimating Sound Transmission Loss

Overall results - The result of all these resonances and coincidences is that the overall behavior of the barrier does not come very close to the mass law except over a limited range at the middle frequencies. A typical Transmission Loss curve shows these effects (Figure 3-2). Estimating the transmission loss of a composite material or system can become complex. Many researchers have investigated and evolved any number of techniques for predicting the sound barrier performance (Figure 3-3 for one example).

Because resonances can significantly reduce the effectiveness of a sound barrier, a material that does not suffer from these is a desirable noise barrier. Since massive limp materials show less degradation due to resonances (they behave more closely to the mass law), the use of lead and loaded plastics has become quite popular in noise control applications. However, Sound Transmission Class (STC) ratings include the effects of resonances so that materials with similar STC ratings can provide similar performance in many applications, unless there are special requirements at the resonant frequency. For example, 5/8" gypsum board (0.4 lb/sq. ft.) has about the same STC as 1/16" lead-vinyl (1.7 lb/sq. ft.) (See Transmission Loss performance in Appendix 4). Thickness of materials affect many material attributes that in turn will change the sound transmission loss or STC of a material. As the thickness increases so does mass and one might predict the performance using the mass law (i.e. each doubling of mass increases transmission loss by 6 dB). However, thickness also changes the material stiffness and internal damping characteristics. As a result, it is recommended that actual test data be used to determine transmission loss performance. A typical example of the complexity is demonstrated in glass (Figure 3-4).

SOME SPECIFIC BARRIER MATERIALS

Probably the most economical and easiest-to-use noise barrier materials are those that are already present in a building. These are, of course, common building materials such as steel, wood, concrete, brick, gypsum board, glass, and plaster. The sound transmission class of some of these materials is shown in Appendix 4. For concrete with a light aggregate, the effect on the sound transmission is equivalent to reducing the thickness of the wall. The lightest aggregate can be equivalent to a reduction of about one-third. Also, when using concrete block, the more porous the block the lower the transmission loss. Consequently, painting concrete block with a sealing paint increases the transmission loss. For dense concrete block, this increase can be as much as 10 dB.

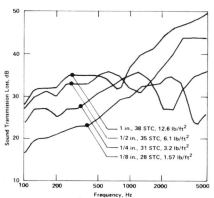

Figure 3-4 - Sound transmission loss for various thickness of glass.

Other materials used as structural components as well as sound barriers include metals, wood, fibrous and cementious boards, glass, stone, and many common artificial materials and composites such as paperboard, vinyl, fiberglass reinforced plastic (FRP), rigid foam (closed cell), roofing, wall coverings, and floor coverings. Some products used as sound absorbers such as slotted concrete blocks and perforated clay tiles have some barrier capability in addition to their role as sound absorbers. Many barriers are combined with absorbing materials. Called "composites," many provide both barrier and absorptive characteristics.

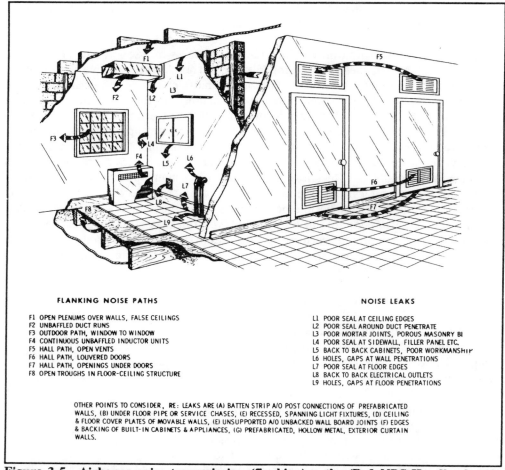

Figure 3-5 - Airborne noise transmission (flanking) paths (Ref. NBS Handbook 119)

All of these materials, when incorporated into a structure, can provide good sound barrier properties. Frequently though, they have windows, doors and penetrations for HVAC, and power or water pipes. These penetrations will significantly affect and many times dramatically reduce the transmission loss (TL) of the barrier. In addition to the average window being the weak link, the mounting is such, or the window is left open, so that the TL performance is degraded even further (Figure 3-5).

A common material that is not generally used for structural purposes but that has high utility for sound barrier applications is lead. Lead is a dense material and is comparatively inexpensive. Also thin lead sheet effectively simulates a limp mass. These considerations make it a very useful barrier material. Usually lead is used in combination with other materials which provide sound absorption, create a floating lead septum away from a vibrating surface, or simply cover up the exposed lead surfaces. The limpness and natural damping of lead means that it does not suffer from the severe TL reducing coincidence dip of the other common materials. The TL characteristics of lead follow fairly closely to the mass law relationship.

Lead is also probably the most used material for adding mass to the well-known plastic materials. However, recent environmental concerns have caused manufacturers to replace lead with other inert high mass materials. These materials offer convenience of use and ease of installation that a rigid sound barrier generally cannot provide. They are generally very flexible and can be hung as curtains around a noisy machine or used as doors between noisy spaces. Complete machine enclosures can be formed with the loaded vinyl simply by providing a frame to hang them on (Figure 3-6).

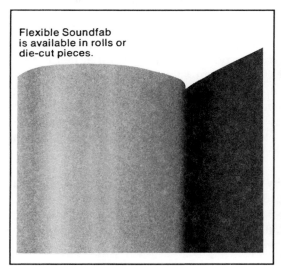

Figure 3-6 - Loaded vinyl materials

Loaded plastics are even made that are transparent so that an operator can see the machine which is enclosed. They are also moldable and can be shaped to cover the outside of any desired surface.

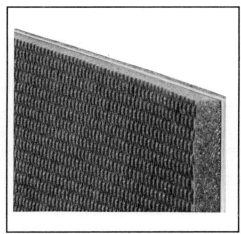

Figure 3-7 - Composite barrier materials

Since these materials are designed to be used as sound barriers, and since sound barriers (especially complete enclosures) are aided by the addition of sound absorbing material to the inside, the obvious next step is to combine lead, loaded vinyl, foam, fiberglass, etc. into composite materials. In addition to a single layer of porous absorber on one side of the barrier material, these products come in multilayered sandwich laminated forms. These sandwich forms combine the acoustical properties of; absorption, a limp sound barrier not rigidly suspended, damped TL properties, and even provide some damping to the outside skin to which they may be attached (Figure 3-7).

Mastic materials are any of a variety of quick drying pasting cements. For sound barrier applications, they are usually a type of dense flexible asphalted product. Their pliability ranges from flexible to semirigid. They are heavyweight products used as sound barrier or damping materials in automobiles, hollow core doors, appliances, etc. Resinated cotton is sometimes added to mastic to provide vibration damping and to avoid direct contact between mastic and other surfaces in certain cases. Like mastics, these products also have pliability ranging from flexible to semirigid and can be used in door or wall cavities, enclosures, etc., to increase the transmission loss of existing structures.

In addition to the sound absorbing spray-on materials, there are also sound barrier types. Spray-on materials are used to increase the sound transmission loss of a system, usually by spraying the product into the cavity of an existing structure. Spray compounds also can reduce the structureborne noise by damping the structure to which they are applied. Spray-on materials effectively stop the sound leaks and increase the acoustic resistance of the cavities into which they are sprayed.

In most applications the structure must be fabricated, applied, connected, etc., and adhesives are the only way. Today there is virtually no construction or assembly material that cannot be bonded with some form of available adhesive. Modern adhesives combine mechanical strength with the ability to function in the heat or cold and resist many of the acids, alkalis, oils, etc. to which they may be exposed. Common adhesives come in solvent based, water based, hot melt, film, and curable liquids. Since they must meet many rigorous demands, it is important that they are utilized properly and the manufacturer's directions are followed carefully.

Just as with adhesives, the form and availability of sealants is also varied. Sealants come in room temperature gunable butyls, hot extruded elastomers, and as tapes with pre-applied pressure sensitive adhesive. Because, as we have seen, the effectiveness of a sound barrier can be significantly reduced by leaks, these sealants perform the vital function of helping to maintain the design performance of a sound barrier assembly.

BARRIER SYSTEMS

Walls, floors, roofs and ceilings are commonly used to contain noise. Their ability to reduce the noise to an acceptable level depends on the following factors:

- Airtightness - Barriers must be acoustically sealed to avoid sound leaks or flanking
- Mass - Doubling mass may increase transmission loss by 6 dB
- Resilient mount - Separate surface materials from structural supports or opposite face
- Absorbent core - When faces are decoupled, sound absorbing core materials are effective

Design of walls and floor/ceiling assemblies for superior sound transmission class (STC) ratings has resulted in a multitude of system designs. Research by major building materials manufacturers has identified the foregoing principals to be significant in attaining practical STC ratings for systems that must also perform other functions, such as fire barriers, structural support, etc. In commercial buildings, where non-load bearing partitions may be used, partition systems composed of 25 ga. drywall steel studs spaced 24" o. c. with gypsum wallboard facings and a core filled with a mineral wool blanket have become the industry standard (Figure 3-8). STC ratings of 35 to 60 have been attained with layered variations. This system is so effective primarily because the steel studs act as a resilient or decoupling mechanism between the gypsumboard faces, which in turn allows the sound absorbing core and increasing thickness of wallboard to increase the STC. Each addition of a layer of wallboard adds approximately 5 STC as does the addition of a sound absorbing blanket. By contrast, standard 2 x 4 wood studs, required for load bearing walls, act as a wall face coupler. Additional layers of wallboard and-

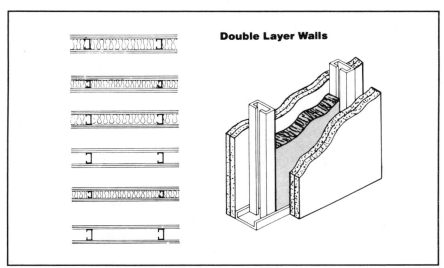

Figure 3-8 - Steel stud partition

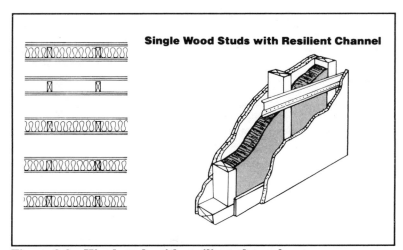

Figure 3-9 - Wood studs with resilient channels

/or sound absorbing blankets are relatively ineffective at increasing the STC until a resilient mount is utilized. Resilient furring channels have become the standard technique in this situation. They are also effective on the ceiling side of floor/ceiling assemblies (Figure 3-9).

Appendix 3 contains a worksheet to calculate the effectiveness of various barrier configurations including composite wall or barrier assemblies containing windows, doors and other penetrations. Appendix 4 contains the sound transmission loss performance characteristics of a wide range of materials and systems of construction.

TEST PROCEDURES FOR SOUND TRANSMISSION LOSS

Laboratory and field tests have been well established for evaluating the noise reduction or sound transmission loss of barriers. In fact, a whole family of test procedures has been established by the American Society of Testing and Materials (ASTM). Committee E-33 on Environmental Acoustics, specifically Subcommittee 02 - Transmission Loss wrote procedure ASTM E-90, the most well known of these procedures. Titled "Standard Test Method for Laboratory Measurement of Airborne Sound Transmission Loss of Building Partitions," the procedure utilizes a source and receiving room with the specimen under test placed in a 9 by 14 foot opening. In essence the two rooms are duplicate reverberation chambers similar to those used for absorption testing. Transmission loss results include frequencies between 125 and 4000 Hz. A single number rating called the Sound Transmission Class (STC) is established according to ASTM E-413 (Figure 3-10). For field measurements, use ASTM E-336. (Note: a more detailed discussion of applicable ASTM test procedures may be found in Appendix 2).

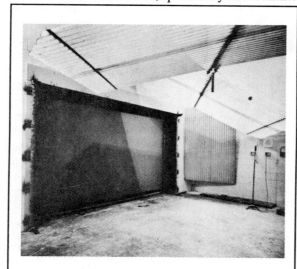

Figure 3-10 - Sound Transmission Loss test. Two identical reverberant chambers are joined with a 9' by 14' opening for test specimen. (ASTM E-90)

DUCT ATTENUATION

Noise that is transmitted down a round or square duct, such as utilized in an Heating, Ventilation and Air Conditioning (HVAC) distribution system, can be reduced substantially. The technique most widely utilized is to line the **inside** of the duct with highly sound-absorbing material. As the sound travels down the duct, it will bounce off the side walls. With a sound-absorbing inside lining, such as glass fiber board, each sound reflection is

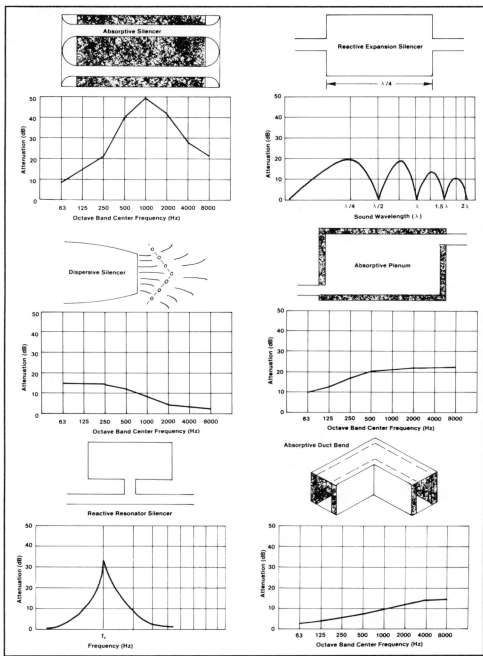

Figure 3-11 - Duct attenuators & silencers

absorbed a little. After a multitude of reflections, most noise has been reduced and is termed "duct attenuation." Duct attenuation is measured in dB per lineal foot. The most widely known test procedure is ASTM E-477. Where it is necessary to attenuate duct noise in a short distance, prefabricated duct attenuators are installed in line with the air duct. These devices are highly efficient sound absorbers, yet exhibit low resistance to air flow down the duct. Sound attenuation can be equivalent to the transmission loss values of many barriers (Figure 3-11). Sound attenuation data for some common duct liners may be found under the appropriate section in Appendix 4.

Transmission through the side wall of air ducts is cause for concern if located near the air moving fans or chillers. In this situation, the duct walls must be good sound barriers. To improve the sound barrier capabilities of sheet metal ducts, additional wraps of an absorbing material covered with a good barrier such as lead or gypsum board may be required. This is a particularly difficult problem in HVAC system noise. There are no easy solutions. While no particular test procedure has been developed for this specific situation, several barrier procedures are adaptable. For field analysis the Noise Reduction (NR) portions of ASTM E-336 may be appropriate.

PIPE NOISE

Noise emanating from liquid flow piping systems is of particular concern in industrial environments. Steam and rapid liquid flow of all types create turbulence in the line at valves, bends and any obstruction. This noise may even set up resonant vibrations that excite adjacent panels or structural supports. Vibration issues are covered in Chapter 5. Quieting pipe noise is primarily a design issue. The key design principal is to keep the flow of liquid smooth and at an even pressure. To reduce turbulence, pipe bends should have a long radius and the inside of the pipe should be smooth. Valves are a particular problem since their purpose is to restrict the flow. However, with proper though potentially costly design, valves can be made quiet. When redesign is not practical, pipe covers constructed of good barrier materials are appropriate. Covering the pipe with a fibrous material will act as both a damper and sound absorber. In most instances, the pipe covering must be combined with a good sound barrier. Again, standard test procedures do not exist though several have been proposed (Figure 3-12).

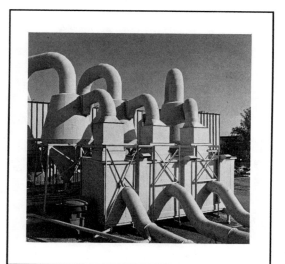

Figure 3-12 - Sound attenuating pipe lagging.

****

Chapter 4 - VIBRATION DAMPING MATERIALS

DAMPING VIBRATIONS

The dynamic resonances and sound barrier properties of a structure are governed primarily by mass, stiffness, and damping. Mass and stiffness were discussed in Chapter 3. Damping is perhaps the most unpredictable and complex property. The word "damping" has been used loosely for many years to denote any number of noise abatement procedures. Frequently used, almost self contradictory phrases such as "damp out the sound in the room" and "use sound damping mounts under the machine" indicate the state of popular confusion among the mechanisms of vibration damping, sound absorption, and vibration isolation.

Part of the difficulty in predicting damping is that there are so many physical mechanisms involved, and any or all of them may be important factors in a particular problem. These physical mechanisms include viscosity, friction (including internal), temperature, shape, acoustic radiation, turbulence, and mechanical and magnetic hysteresis.

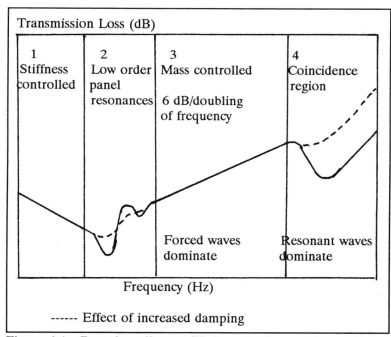

Figure 4-1 - Damping effect on TL for a flat homogenous panel

While the prediction and analysis of damping may be an elusive thing, the benefits to be obtained from adding damping to the structure can yield big rewards. Damping reduces the amplitude of vibrations at resonant frequencies. These reduced vibrations, in turn, result in reduced sound radiation, lowered structural stress, and reduced fatigue problems. Damping is particularly helpful when dealing with noise radiated from the free vibrations caused by impacts between parts of a structure, such as loose parts striking metal chutes. Structureborne sound is also reduced (i.e. transmission of vibrational energy along the structure is reduced). In addition, the transmission loss performance of a barrier is increased in the resonance region but more particularly at, and above, the critical coincidence frequency (Figure 4-1).

More recently, it has been shown that most structural materials, in actual applications, do not behave exactly as measured under laboratory conditions. They do not follow the mass law when the material is stiffened by reinforcing ribs or stiffening swages. The result is a complex set of responses that can be reduced by adding damping to the structure, thereby reducing sound radiation.

Measuring Damping

Damping effectiveness is generally expressed in terms of dimensionless numbers such as loss factor, damping ratio, or percent of critical damping (Figure 4-2). Typical methods for testing the damping properties of a material involve measuring the decay rate of a freely suspended panel, or measuring the band width at the half power point of a simple beam resonance.

While all materials exhibit some natural damping, the amount in most metals is too low to be of any practical significance. Even lead, which is often thought of as being highly damped, only has a loss factor of approximately 0.001. To have any significance, the composite loss factor of a system should be about 0.05 or higher. Care must be taken when choosing a damping material, as some of the high damping synthetic rubbers have material loss factors as high as 5 at certain frequencies and temperatures, whereas the composite loss factors of realistic structural systems rarely go higher than 0.5.

Types of Treatment

The two major types of damping are free layer and constrained layer, and some materials could be considered a combination of both. The free layer treatment consists of a single layer of viscoelastic material applied to the base structure, and the bending vibration of the base material induces extensional deformation of the viscoelastic layer. The constrained layer treatment could consist of either two layers of material added to the existing structure: a layer of viscoelastic material, and a layer of relatively stiff material, usually sheet metal, or it could consist of the structural material itself with the viscoelastic material sandwiched between two layers of sheet metal.

In either case, the bending vibration of the structure induces shear-deformation in the viscoelastic material due to the constraint provided on the boundary of the viscoelastic layer by the two layers of stiff material. The vibrational energy loss is due to the heat generated by the cyclic deformation of the viscoelastic material. But because of the different deformation inducing mechanisms of the two treatments, a damping material that provides good results in one treatment will usually not be effective in the other. In general, effective free layer materials are comparatively stiff and must be applied in thick layers, while effective constrained layer materials are relatively compliant and may be quite efficient in very thin layers.

The effectiveness of layered damping treatments depends on a number of variables. Base structure properties of importance are thickness, inherent damping, resonance frequency, wavelength of vibration at resonance, modulus of elasticity, and density. The constraining layer properties of importance are thickness, modulus of elasticity, and density. The important properties of the viscoelastic material used in the treatment are thickness, density, shear modulus, and material loss factor. The latter two properties of the viscoelastic material are functions of both temperature and frequency. Therefore, it is important to have an accurate description of the modulus and loss factor as functions of temperature and frequency in order to accurately evaluate the effectiveness of the material's damping treatment. Because the properties of the viscoelastic material are temperature and frequency sensitive, the amount of damping provided by a layered viscoelastic damping treatment will also vary with temperature and frequency. It is essential that a damping treatment be properly designed for it to be effective.

By combining viscoelastic material technology and vibration theory, it is possible to develop design procedures for predicting the performance of several types of damping treatments applied to structures. This approach can be demonstrated for simple beams, but it can and has been applied to more complex systems such as plates and stiffened structures (Figure 4-3). The analysis has been found to be a powerful design tool, allowing the elimination of much of the guesswork that has been associated with the "cut and try" approach to structural damping.

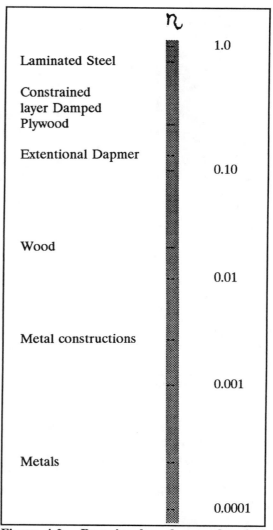

Figure 4-2 - **Damping loss factor of typical materials.**

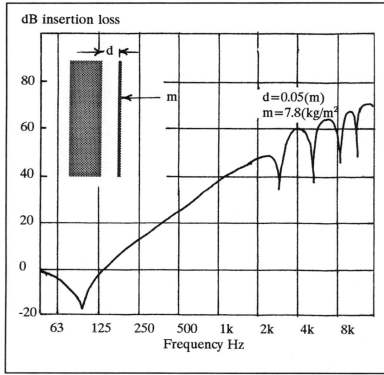

Figure 4-3 - Insertion loss of close fitting laminated steel shield.

Common Damping Materials

High damping has been designed into some special metals, but vibration damping usually involves the application of viscoelastic materials such as rubbers or plastics to the vibrating member. The most suitable substances for this are the high molecular weight polymers.

Materials intended solely for the purpose of vibration damping are available in semifluid form for application with a spray gun or trowel. A few are soft enough after drying to indent with the thumbnail, but most of the height effective compositions are hard and seemingly brittle at room temperatures. Damping materials are also available in the form of pre-cured or extruded sheets or rolls which can be glued or heat bonded onto the structure. Other materials can be supplied already laminated into a metal sheet or coil. Some even come with a magnetic backing so that they can be fastened simply by laying pieces on the part to be damped.

Bonding

In all of the available types of damping materials, it is essential that energy is transferred effectively between the vibrating panel and the damping material. For this to occur, the surfaces must be securely bonded together, and since the bonding agent becomes part of the system, its physical properties are also important. Generally, however, the bonding agent is either built into the material that is to be sprayed or troweled on, or can be purchased from the supplier of the damping material. Obviously a secure application of the damping material will include a thorough cleansing of all grease and dirt from the surface to be damped.

Constrained Layer Materials

Currently the technology exists to provide constrained layer damping materials in most metals, wood and wood products, plastic, and fiber reinforced plastic sheets. The viscoelastic materials can be supplied in a form that could be added to an existing structure by post laminating. Or, the structural material itself can be supplied with the viscoelastic material pre-laminated into the middle.

Post Laminated Constrained Layer Systems

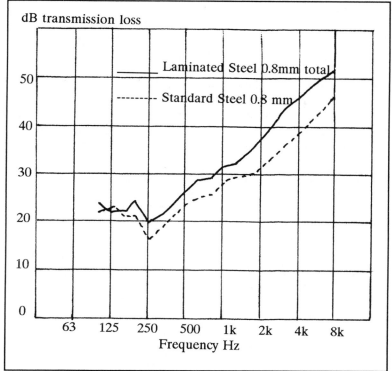

Figure 4-4 - TL of laminated and regular steel

The simplest form of a post laminated constrained layer system is aluminum or steel foil with a viscoelastic material. The viscoelastic layer may be a pressure sensitive adhesive sheet. These sheets can be easily cut to shape and pressed onto the surface of the structure. The pressure sensitive adhesive must be formulated to provide the correct viscoelastic properties, as well as to maintain the bond between the structure and the foil.

The viscoelastic inner layer, when used as a pressure sensitive adhesive, can be supplied so that it can join two or more structural materials. The inner layer in this case would be a transfer film between two release papers or coatings on two sides of a carrier material.

The viscoelastic material, when used as a solid layer, can be bonded with an adhesive in between the structural elements (taking care that the characteristics of the adhesive do not detract form the effectiveness of the inner layer). Or, in the case of fiber reinforced plastic, the viscoelastic material can be bonded into the system by the polymer matrix as it cures. The inner layer, in this particular case, must be protected from the catalyst in the polymer matrix or it could harden the viscoelastic material and render it ineffective.

Pre-laminated Metals

These materials are usually available in coils with overall thickness from 0.020" to 0.125" weighing up to 20,000 lbs. They are more commonly available in sheets with overall thicknesses from 0.020" to 0.25", and sheet sizes up to 4 ft. by 8 ft. Sometimes the fabricator can be given pre-cut blanks which could have originated from coil or sheet laminate. The metals in the laminates can be any commercially available metal such as steel, aluminum, copper, etc. These laminates can be fabricated as regular materials, provided the supplier's recommendations for tool adjustments and joining are followed. Some examples of typical loss factors for pre-laminated flat steel systems are shown in Figure 4-4.

Highly damped laminates are used in applications where impact and boundary excited vibration is important. Examples in the automotive industry include oil pans and rocker arm covers. In the appliance industry damped laminates are used to quiet dish washer cabinets. In the manufacturing industry these materials are used in busses, trucks, machinery, computers, military vehicles and equipment, lawn care equipment, generators and compressors. A new and exciting application is in the construction of floor systems in residential and lightweight commercial buildings. Damped plywood and cementious board composites are applied as the subfloor using conventional installation techniques. Tests have shown a marked improvement of the impact noise due to footfalls for both the source and receiver positions.

Highly damped laminates are also used when increased transmission loss is required. Damped laminates improve the barrier characteristics of the system at resonance frequencies and at the critical coincidence frequency. Examples of these applications would be the dash panel on a car or the engine bulkhead on buses, trucks, ships and buildings.

FREE LAYER DAMPING MATERIALS

Homogenous Materials

Used for damping at or around room temperature on thin sheet metal surfaces that have little or no stiffness added in the form of swages or ribs, homogenous materials often are low budget materials made from limestone filled tar and bitumen compounds. These materials must be used in thick layers (over twice as thick as the metal structure) to be effective. They are heavy and usually difficult to handle at low temperatures due to their brittleness. These materials are usually bonded to the sheet metal using heat fusion by passing them through an oven.

The higher-performance (and more expensive) materials in this group are mica filled polymer compounds which are much lighter and can be made fire resistant to meet the safety needs of the computer and appliance markets. These materials are generally bonded to the substrate using pressure sensitive adhesive systems such as acrylic or rubber compounds coated to the underside of the damping sheet and protected by a silicone coated release paper. To install the damping sheet, the release paper is removed and pressure applied to the damping sheet to activate the adhesive. The manufacturer must be careful in selecting this adhesive because if it is too soft, it will destroy the acoustical efficiency of the damping sheet. Conversely, if it is too stiff, the pressure required to make it stick will be unacceptably high.

Both types of damping sheets can be supplied with either a polyurethane foam or a fibrous material on top to make a combined structural/damping/sound absorbing system.

Nonhomogeneous Materials

A combination of all the damping materials above, nonhomogeneous materials are free layer systems that are added to the structure after fabrication. They have damping compounds on the upper surface which absorb energy in extension and compression. They are also constrained layer systems in that they rely on the multiple layers in their construction to absorb the vibration energy in shear.

Similar to free layer materials, nonhomogeneous materials can be heat bonded in paint ovens or applied using pressure sensitive adhesives which make them a fundamental part of the damping system.

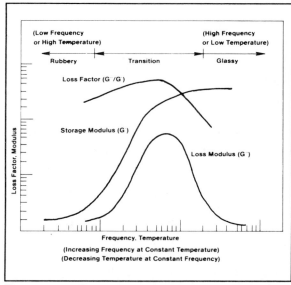

Figure 4-5 - Dependance of storage modulus, loss modulus and loss factor on temperature and frequency for an elastomeric vibration damping material

Effects of Temperature and Thickness

Most damping materials exhibit similar dependence on temperature. At low temperatures, the materials are glassy or very hard. At higher temperatures the materials become soft and rubbery. In effect, they function effectively only in the middle of the temperature range (Figure 4-5).

To overcome part of the temperature limitation, most manufacturers have been able to design polymers so that most of the temperature range normally encountered is acceptable. Typical curves depict the temperature dependence of a family of damping materials. With data supplied in this manner, it is only necessary to know the operating temperature range to be encountered. One may then select the appropriate members of the family. Other materials take advantage of the temperature dependence of damping material and start with a glass-type base that is hard at normal temperatures. By starting with this material, good damping can be achieved in the 1000 to 1200 degree F range.

When applying mastic dampers, there is considerable advantage in determining regions of large amplitude and maximum stress panel vibration, and then concentrating the material at that location in greater thickness, rather than using uniform weight material coverage. The reason is made clear by the illustration (Figure 4-6) where the effectiveness of a typical mastic damper is plotted as a function of thickness ratio. Note that the loss factor of a panel treated with a mastic layer depends on the thickness ratio between the treatment layer and the panel, rather than on the thickness itself. Also, the approximate square law dependence on thickness ratio favors application of all the treatment on one side of the panel, rather than dividing the weight of the mastic between two layers on opposite sides.

Significant weight and cost economy can be realized by concentrating the damping mastic in the antinodal vibration areas where maximum stress occurs. However, information about the vibration nodal pattern is generally not available and full coverage of the panel is necessary. Full coverage of the entire vibrating panel will assure that the motion of every possible vibration node of the panel will be coupled to the damping material, and its energy will be dissipated. If material is applied in a patch without knowledge of or regard to the vibration patterns of high-frequency modes, some of the high-frequency tones are almost certain to remain undamped. Caution, be sure material is applied to the edges of flat panels.

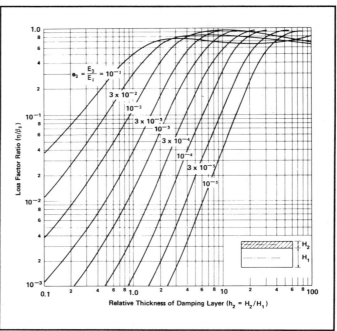

Figure 4-6 - Dependence of loss factor of a panel on viscoelastic layer thickness and elastic modulus.

The problem of how much damping material is needed, or how effective a damping treatment is required in a given application is best determined experimentally. Use a few general rules and simple computations to guide a trial-and-error determination.

With only a few trials, using progressively less effective treatments, it is easy to locate the point of diminishing returns where the effect of further damping of resonant-noise components is masked by noises from other sources. By this procedure, the minimum damping capacity that will provide the maximum noise reduction is established.

Acceptable damping is commonly defined as achieving a composite loss factor of 0.05 over the frequency and temperature range of interest. This would imply that a typical steel structure with a loss factor of 0.001 has had its damping increased by a factor of 20. In aerospace and similar applications, a minimum composite loss factor of 0.1 may be required.

It should also be noted that the cost advantages of attaining high damping with homogeneous materials of damping foils on thin sheet metal diminish rapidly as the thickness of the metal to be damped increases. This is because of the extra layers needed, or the increased thickness of these layers needed for high damping with thick plates. In such cases, constrained layer viscoelastic materials, in very thin sheets, provide far better damping with a substantial advantage in cost and thickness of damping treatment.

SUMMARY

Damping is a particularly effective means to quiet noise at the source. By adding a damping material to a vibrating panel or placing vibrating equipment on a damping pad, the resulting noise levels may be dramatically reduced. Two types of damping are called free layer and constrained layer damping. Vibrational energy losses are due to heat generated by cyclic deformation of viscoelastic materials. Damping materials have quite different characteristics with a change in temperature, humidity and age. Designs take into account a number of material variables including thickness, inherent damping, resonance, frequency, modulus of elasticity and density.

****

Chapter 5 - SILENCERS

SILENCER TYPES

Silencers come in many shapes and sizes and most all of them can be classified into four types: reactive, dissipative, absorptive, and dispersive or diffusive. Reactive silencers do not use sound absorbing materials but instead employ geometric design principles. An example is the Helmholtz resonator. Absorptive silencers use conventional sound absorbing materials. Dissipative silencers utilize flow resistance to reduce flow velocity. Dispersive or diffusive silencers reduce noise by preventing its generation. By diffusing high-velocity turbulent gas flow to a lower velocity less turbulent flow, less noise is generated. Some silencers will combine the action of two or more of the four types within one envelope. Other functions such as water separation, filtering, spark arresting, or heat recovery may be integrated into the silencer as well (Figure 5-1).

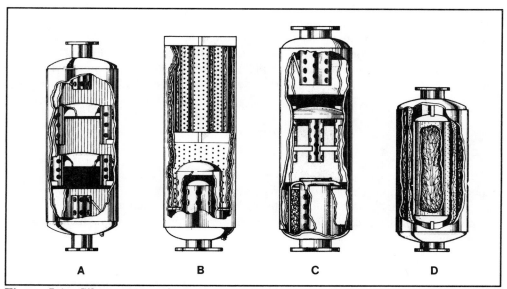

Figure 5-1 - Silencer examples

Reactive and Dissipative Silencers

The simplest form of a reactive silencer is a plain expansion chamber in the ductwork carrying the sound. At each change in the cross-sectional area of the duct, the impedance change causes a reflection of the sound waves. This reflection added to the subsequent destructive interference with the incoming sound results in a noise reduction along the duct.

Another simple form is a chamber attached to the side of the duct via a hole or holes in the duct wall or via a short pipe or pipes between the duct and chamber. A ducted chamber such as this works on the principle of a Helmholtz resonator. A side branch pipe may be attached to the side of the duct. This works on the principle of a tuned organ pipe. Long large pipes absorb low frequency and small short pipes absorb higher frequencies of sound. However, because of the way these silencers perform, they only have good noise reduction over a narrow range of frequencies. Complex designs have been developed, however, that offer broad frequency performance. Reactive silencers find their greatest use in silencing pulsating gas flows such as engine intakes, exhausts, blowers, etc.

Dissipative silencers utilize flow resistance to supplement the reactive silencer qualities. This is obtained by incorporating perforations or ports in the flow passage tubes so that main flow passage resistance is not increased.

Absorptive Silencers

Absorptive silencers are devices which use the sound absorptive properties of a porous material to absorb the sound on its passage through the device. Probably the simplest absorptive silencer is the common lined duct. Lining the inside walls of a duct with sound absorbing material can provide a silencer of almost any desired length. To predict the sound attenuation performance of a lined duct, the sound attenuation in dB per foot is:

$$Attenuation(dB/ft) = 12.6 \times \alpha^{1.4} \times \frac{P}{S}$$

P = perimeter of the duct inside the lining (inches)
S = cross sectional area of the duct inside the lining (inches squared)
α = Sabine absorption coefficient of the lining material obtained from laboratory measurements.

This equation provides good agreement with measurements for the lower frequencies. However, for the middle to higher frequencies, the calculated value of noise reduction is below that actually achieved for the first several feet. In addition, this equation does not account for line-of-sight propagation through the duct of the higher frequency sound (line-of-sight transmitted sound does not impinge on the lining and is not absorbed). Depending on the size of the duct, the practical limit for high frequency sound attenuation is about 10 dB, with the limit approaching the predicted value as the frequency is lowered. High-frequency performance of a lined duct can be improved by lining bends in the ductwork or inserting some additional lined bends.

Another simple form of combination reactive and absorptive silencer is a lined sound absorbing plenum. The attenuation provided by such a plenum can be determined by the empirical expression:

$$Attenuation(dB) = -10\log[S_c\cos\Theta\pi d^2 + 1 - \frac{\alpha}{\alpha S_w}]$$

α = absorption coefficient of the lining (frequency dependant)
S_c = plenum exit area (sq. ft.)
S_w = plenum wall area (sq. ft.)
d = distance between entrance and exit (ft.)
Θ = the angle of incidence at the exit, i.e., the angle d makes with the normal to the exit opening (degrees).

The sound attenuation characteristics of plenums and lined ducts can be increased by introducing additional sound absorbing surfaces which increase the path length and eliminate the line-of-sight problems of plain ducts.

For ease of installation, and for the benefit of predicted sound attenuation performance, many sizes and styles of prepackaged silencers are available. For heavier duty applications pipeline silencers offering more rugged construction are also available.

Dispersive Silencers

Aerodynamic noise resulting from gas or vapor flow through an orifice or control valve is a predominant source of noise in piping systems. Dispersion or diffusion type silencers are pressure reducing devices. They fit in the piping downstream from the restriction and reduce the pressure ratio across the restriction. The result is low noise levels. These devices can be designed as a cage surrounding the control valve or as attachments behind the valve. Other diffuser type silencers for gases exhausting to the atmosphere include combination absorptive-reactive-absorptive-velocity reduction type silencers.

Low-frequency Silencers

Low-frequency noise control of reciprocating engines, rotary blowers, vacuum pumps, compressors, and vents is normally accomplished with standard reactive, and other, silencers. These usually involve relatively high pressure drops, low mass flows, and maximum noise reductions in the 125 and 250 Hz bands.

Stack-insert Silencers

Another type of low frequency noise problem, usually in the 125 to 250 Hz band, may occur in industrial exhaust stacks for paint-spray booths or foundries. Here the principal noise source may be the fan at an essentially discrete tone corresponding to the fan blade passage frequency. Again airflows may be relatively high and permissible pressure drops very low.

One solution to this type of problem is the stack-insert silencer that is designed to drop into the stack itself. This type of silencer is considerably less expensive than a normal silencer because the walls of the stack form the shell of the silencer.

Blowdown and Line Silencers

Blowdown silencers and line silencers utilize the same internal components and the same absorptive/reactive design for attenuation of high intensity noise. Air, steam, or other gases, with flows that can exceed 1,000,000 CFM, enter the silencers through nozzles designed to withstand cyclic, dynamic, and thermal stresses. An energy dissipating inlet diffuser transforms the noise spectrum into easier-to-attenuate high frequencies within an acoustically-lined plenum which prevents shell radiation and noise leakage. Floating modules of perforated tubes packed with sound absorptive material are the major silencing elements in the assembly.

Blowdown silencers, available in sizes ranging from 12 inches to 12 feet in diameter, are recommended for silencing noise generated by compressor blowoffs; boiler start-up and purge systems; relief, safety and snort valves; steam ejectors; or any other high-intensity vent generated noise.

Line silencers can be coupled directly to bypass the control valves for reducing in-line noise of pressurized, continuous flowing gases. They can also be applied to the inlet or discharge of centrifugal compressors and to the inlet of gas turbines. They are available in all sizes consistent with these applications.

Duct Silencers

Tubular or rectangular duct silencers with capacities ranging from 100 to over 400,000 CFM are recommended for reducing intake or discharge noises from large fans, gas turbines and blowers. The high ratio of insertion loss per foot of length is due to an absorptive area comprised of multiple ducts lined with airfoil-shaped perforated metal backed with sound absorptive material. Entrances and exits are formed to provide low flow resistance and pressure loss.

Note that a simple version of a duct silencer is a sound absorbent lined duct. For air handling ducts, sound attenuation is based on sound pressure levels measured in a reverberation room after sound passes through a 10 foot specimen and enters the reverberation room as outlined in ASTM Method E-477. Duct attenuation is presented in dB per lineal foot of duct liner at octave band frequencies between 125 and 4000 Hz for a whole array of duct sizes and insulation thicknesses by several manufacturers. Values will increase for every 90 degree bend in the duct. Air velocity and direction usually have little effect on attenuation, although most testing is done at 1200 FPM air velocity.

ACTIVE DUCT SILENCERS

The concept of reducing and possibly canceling the sound field of a source by using interfering sound waves from another source 180 degrees out of phase is an old concept. When the latest in digital computers is applied to the problem, it becomes an exciting new method of noise control. Called Active Attenuation, Active Noise Control, or more precisely, Digital Sound Cancellation, this method of noise control uses the latest advances in digital signal processing to achieve significant reduction in unwanted noise (Figure 5-2).

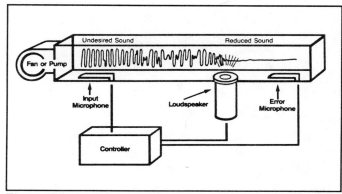

Figure 5-2 - Active duct silencer

Figures 5-2 and 5-3 show a digital sound cancellation system configured to be a duct silencer. An input microphone probe tube measures the noise in the duct. This signal is sent to a digital controller which inverts the fan noise so that it is 180 degrees out of phase. The controller also reshapes the fan sound spectrum so that it is more pleasing to the ear. The output of the controller, which is out of phase with the noise coming down the duct, is boosted by an amplifier and put into the duct with a loudspeaker module. This secondary noise source cancels the fan noise. An error microphone is used to adjust the computer model so that the system performs at its optimum efficiency (Figure 5-3).

There are many practical uses for sound cancellation. Commercially available active systems are available as duct silencers and ear protection headphones. Systems for other applications, such as active vibration, electronic mufflers, and small area cancellation are under development but are many years from becoming practical (Figure 5-4).

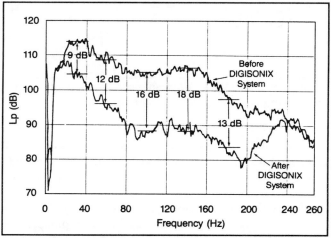

Figure 5-3 - Active silencer broadband reduction (Example courtesy Digisonix)

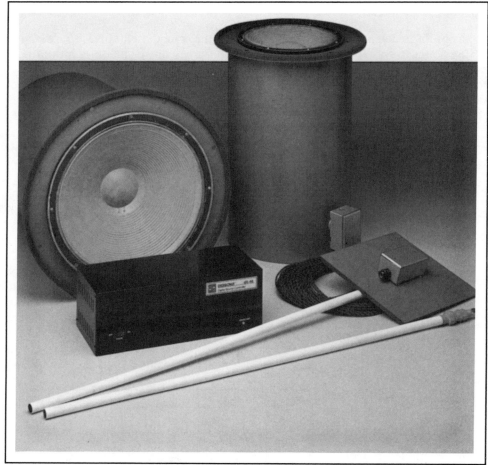

Figure 5-4 - Active duct silencer components including digital controller, acoustic sensing tube, duct access plate and speakers.

When installed in a duct, active attenuation offers excellent low frequency attenuation with near zero pressure drop. The speakers are located outside the duct and can be protected with flexible isolation membranes resulting in minimal pressure drop and regenerated noise.

To date, active duct silencers manufactured by Noise Control Association (NCA) members have been successfully used on fans, vacuum pumps, rotary blowers, and stationary engines (Figure 5-5).

Active/Passive Duct Silencers - Active attenuation can be combined with passive silencers filled with mineral or glass fiber wool. These new "active passive" hybrid silencers attenuate

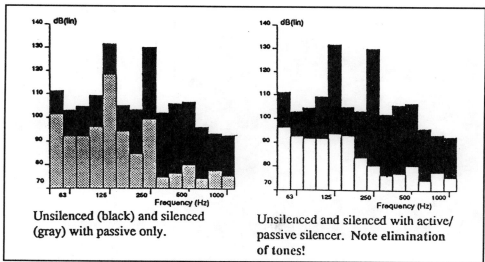

Figure 5-5 - Comparison of active and passive silencers

a broader band of noise (Figure 5-6) with less pressure drop than more conventional approaches. The active portion of the silencer works on the low frequency fan tones and broadband noise while the passive portion of the silencer works on the medium and high frequency noise (Figure 5-7). Active/passive silencers are particularly well-suited for large vane-axial fans since they have a higher frequency content than most other fan types.

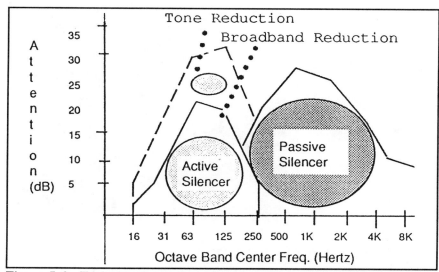

Figure 5-6 - Typical active and passive duct silencer attenuations.

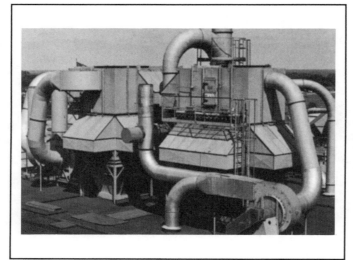

Figure 5-7 - Active silencer on baghouse fan

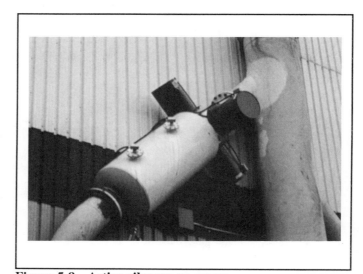

Figure 5-8 - Active silencer on pump

****

Chapter 6 - VIBRATION ISOLATION MATERIALS

TYPES OF VIBRATION ISOLATION MATERIALS

The definition of <u>vibration isolation</u> is the separation, or isolation, of the vibratory forces or motion of one object from another. This is generally accomplished by inserting a flexible material between the driving object and the driven object. Such materials, if sufficiently flexible, will transmit little of the vibrational forces to the driven object. Vibration isolators with little damping are capable of extreme reduction of vibration transmission at the higher frequencies but they permit a great transmission of vibration at the resonant frequency of the system. The addition of damping will limit the response at the resonant frequency but may also reduce the isolation capability at the higher frequencies.

There are two types of vibration isolation applications. The first type is designed to reduce the transmission of vibratory forces from a piece of equipment to the foundation on which it is mounted. The vibration isolation of reciprocating engines, large fans, electric motors, etc., are examples of this type of isolation application. The second type of vibration isolation application is designed to reduce the transmission of vibration velocity or amplitude to the piece of sensitive equipment that is mounted on the floor or to another structural member. The mounting of an optical bench on a massive table which rests on large vibration isolators is an example of this application type.

Some typical materials used for vibration isolators are elastomers, elastomeric foam, cork, felt, fiberglass boards, and steel in such forms as springs, pads, cables, etc. The essential features of vibration isolators are a resilient load-supporting member (stiffness) and energy-dissipating mechanism (damping). In certain types of isolators, the stiffness and damping functions are provided by a single element as in the case of elastomers, elastomeric foam, glass fiber boards, wire mesh, and wire cable isolators. Other types of isolators may employ separate, distinct means of providing stiffness and damping, as in the case of relatively undamped springs used with auxiliary damping elements such as viscous dashpots, coulomb (dry-friction) dampers, and capillary or orifice flow-restriction dampers
(Figure 6-1).

All too often vibrating equipment is mounted on lightweight partitions or floors. Most vibration elements are designed with the concept that the mount is an infinite mass of perfect rigidity. The result is that natural vibration tendencies form a secondary fundamental resonance thereby negating the potential attenuation. Care in the design and selection of the elasticity of the mount are complex issues (Figure 6-2).

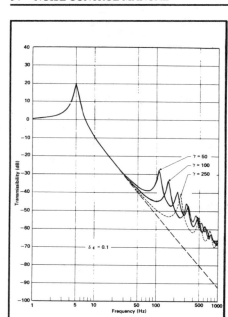

Fig. 6-1 - Simple mounting transmissibility

Shock Isolation

The technology and hardware of shock isolation is different from vibration isolation. A soft resilient spring, such as those used for vibration isolation, may permit much of a shock pulse to be transmitted to the member we wish to protect.

Vibration relates to the steady state, oscillatory motion of a piece of shaking equipment whereas a shock pulse is a substantial disturbance characterized by rise and decay of acceleration in a short period of time.

A shock isolator is a resilient support that isolates a system from a shock pulse. Such isolators are characterized by a long stroke which allows dissipation of energy over a long period of time.

Some Specific Vibration Isolation Materials

The common materials utilized for vibration isolation, such as cork, felt, glass fiber, or elastomers, offer a wide choice to fit most requirements. The main differences between these materials are their stiffness, or natural frequency characteristics, and the amount of damping each can provide. However, the selection of the particular material is usually based on such non-vibration-oriented requirements as resistance to chemicals, tear strength, abrasion resistance, cost, lateral stability, and load capacity. For example, natural rubber has good isolation characteristics and fair temperature dependent properties, but does not age well and does not have the resistance to chemicals possessed by some of the synthetics. Glass fiber which has been prestressed and compressed to high densities provides an effective vibration isolation system for floors of large buildings. Floating floor systems can be effective isolators, protecting sensitive instruments from building structural vibration, or preventing equipment vibrations from being transmitted to the building structure. Glass fiber pads are also used as unit isolators for machinery mountings.

Cork pads, which consist of natural cork granules compressed and steam baked to form slabs of the desired density, have fine aging characteristics and are particularly suitable for isolating concrete foundations.

Felt pads are used for applications in which an isolation material with good cementing characteristics is important. Felt has found widespread use in the textile machinery field and is generally recommended when machinery movement or rebound must be closely controlled.

TRANSMISSIBILITY AND DAMPING

The two characteristics of a vibration isolator that define its effectiveness are transmissibility and damping. Damping is an energy absorbing process and applies when damping is added to an isolator. The principal function of damping in an isolator is to limit the transmissibility of the isolator at the system resonant frequency. Transmissibility is the ability of the isolator to transmit or attenuate the vibratory force or motion from the driving object to the driven object. Transmissibility can refer to the transmission of force, velocity, acceleration, and the like. The curves shown in Figure 6-2 indicate the amount of vibration isolation provided for driving frequencies which are greater than $\sqrt{2}$ times f_o where f_o is the natural resonant frequency of the system with isolator. For driving frequencies less than $\sqrt{2}$ times f_0, the isolator becomes an amplifier, when the driving frequency equals resonant frequency ($f/f_o = 1$).

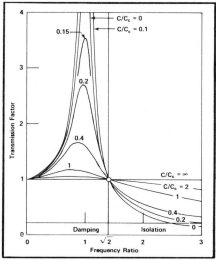

Fig. 6-2 - Transmissibility for a vibration isolation system with viscous damping.

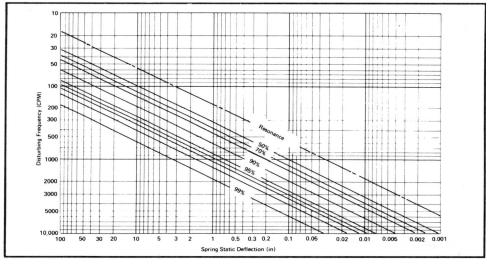

Figure 6-3 - Resonance frequency and percent isolation versus static deflection

Another means of presenting the transmissibility of a linear isolator is through the static deflection. Since the system natural frequency and the static deflection each depend on the stiffness of the isolator, these relationships can be compared, with the result

$$f_o = 1/2\pi \sqrt{g/d}$$

where g is the acceleration due to gravity and d is the deflection of the isolator under a static load. The curves shown in Figure 6-3 show percent isolation versus static deflection and driving frequency for any undamped single degree of freedom isolator. Since these curves hold for any ideal or linear constant stiffness isolator, all that is necessary is to be able to determine the static deflection of an isolator. Read from the chart the percent reduction in vibration for a given driving frequency. Note the lack of any parameter for the isolator in the above equation. This chart is useful to the design engineer as a quick reference for determining how much deflection should be allowed for when isolating a particular piece of equipment.

Harder pads are formed by impregnating layer upon layer of woven cotton duck with natural or synthetic rubber. This is an extremely tough product that is particularly suited to applications where alignment must be maintained. Typical applications are drop hammer anvil pads, printing press column supports, bridge roadway bearing pads, and craneway supports.

Perhaps the most commonly used isolator materials are the elastomers. Elastomers can be molded in many different configurations or materials, including natural rubber, neoprene, butyl, silicone, and a number of combinations of each (Figure 6-4). In addition, various degrees of damping, shape, load-deflection characteristics, and transmissibility characteristics can be designed into elastomeric isolators. The natural damping of elastomers is also useful in preventing problems at resonance that are difficult to restrain with coil springs.

From a standpoint of shock isolation, elastomers offer some advantages because they can generally absorb shock energy per unit weight to a greater extent than other forms of isolator systems.

In addition to these features, elastomeric isolators can be formed so as to provide good lateral stability whereas steel springs generally require some form of stabilizing housing. Elastomeric mounts can also be fabricated that provide comparable vibration isolation characteristics simultaneously in both the horizontal and vertical directions. The felt and foam pads do not suffer from stability problems since they are utilized in a configuration where the height of the isolator is much less than the width.

Elastomers are also produced as pads and frequently have a wafflelike or ribbed surface. These designs provide good gripping surfaces which act to prevent sloping of the mounted machinery in the absence of bolts. In addition, the ribbing controls lateral/vertical stiffness ratio and provides a space for the material to expand when under a compressive load. If a softer spring constant is required, these pads can be stacked to increase the static deflection. The total deflection is simply the product of the number of pads times the deflection of a single pad.

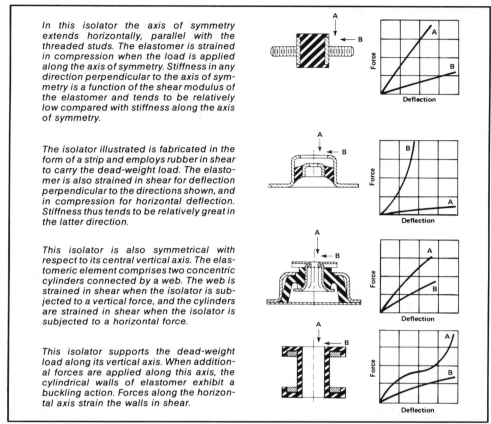

Fig. 6-4 - **Typical elastomeric vibration isolators and their force-deflection curves**

As a general rule, pads are used for eliminating bolting, for minor vibration problems, or for other non-critical applications.

Springs

A common form of vibration isolator is the coil spring. Springs may be loaded in tension, but it is frequently more convenient to load them in compression. The equipment is set up on the springs with a pilot to locate the springs relative to the equipment. Any required auxiliary devices such as leveling or snubbing can be added without much regard to the spring design.

Spring isolator design consists of one or more helical coil springs which are piloted in end caps and contain a central bolt which serves as the tie-in to the equipment. Among the advantages of coil springs are the relatively great freedom in obtaining the necessary stiffness characteristics and freedom from drift or creep. Coil springs are used in vibration isolators primarily for the isolation of low-frequency vibration. Consequently, the coil springs must usually have relatively great static deflection (Figure 6-5).

One of the disadvantages of coil springs is that they possess virtually no damping. Therefore, transmissibility at resonance is extremely high. Coil springs also allow high-frequency surges to get through them and to enter into the sensitive equipment which is being protected. They also are a transmission path for high frequency vibration, which results in an excessively noisy product.

To overcome the disadvantages of little or no damping in coil springs, friction dampers can be designed in parallel with the load carrying spring. These types of isolators are widely used in practice. Another way of adding damping to a spring is by using an air chamber with an orifice for metering the air flow. For applications in which all metal isolators are desired because of temperature extremes or other environmental factors, damping can be added to a load carrying spring by use of metal mesh inserts.

In order to overcome the problem of high frequency noise transmission, one or both ends of the spring can be fitted with elastomeric pads. Conventionally, the pad is attached to the bottom of the spring assembly, which offers the additional advantage of providing a non-slip surface which frequently eliminates the need to bolt the isolator to the floor.

The selection of springs involves consideration of their load-carrying capacities (in terms of stressor or excessive deflections), and where such springs carry vertical loads in compression, their lateral stability. Free-standing helical compression springs must have a large enough coil diameter so that the springs do not buckle sideward under load. Where space limitations do no permit the use of large diameters, a stabilizing housing for the spring must be used.

Another way in which steel is utilized as a vibration isolator is in a coiled cable configuration. These isolators are stable mounting assemblies of stranded stainless steel wire ropes formed between metal retainers. They are used to attenuate vibration and to provide shock protection. Inherent damping of the isolator, which is particularly important for motion control at resonance, is provided by flexure hysteresis. Damping characteristics are related to the strain applied to the isolator. Large motions are highly damped, whereas small amplitude motion is relatively undamped with the isolator appearing to act as a pure spring. The cable can be wound in a helical fashion between two metal bars to assure reliable shock and vibration control. As a base mount, center of gravity mount, and even in cantilevered mounting, coiled cable can provide effective protection in compression, tension, shear, or roll.

Another form of steel vibration isolator, developed primarily for heavy-duty applications where severe shock forces are encountered, utilizes wire mesh as the isolation element. They are recommended for protecting equipment mounted aboard a ship or in vehicular installations. These shock and vibration mounts are fabricated with all-metal resilient cushions for lifetime performance. The high inherent damping qualities provide rapid elimination of shock forces with no severe rebound which often causes more damage than the initial force itself. The non-linear spring rate insures both vibration isolation in a wide working range and overload capacity to withstand shocks as great as 100 g. Within the rated load capacity of each mount, the natural frequency varies inversely with the static load between about 14 - 22 Hz. Multi-directional attenuation and rapid decay of shock pulses without severe rebound is supplemented by isolation at higher exciting frequencies to provide equipment protection.

Resilient cushions are fabricated of stainless steel wire. Exposure to oil, water, solvents, salt water, dust, dirt, and extreme temperatures have no ill effect on the performance of these mounts (Figures 6-5 and 6-6).

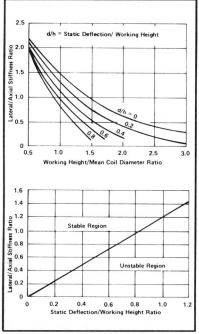

Fig. 6-5 - Helical springs - Ratio of lateral to axial stiffness and stability

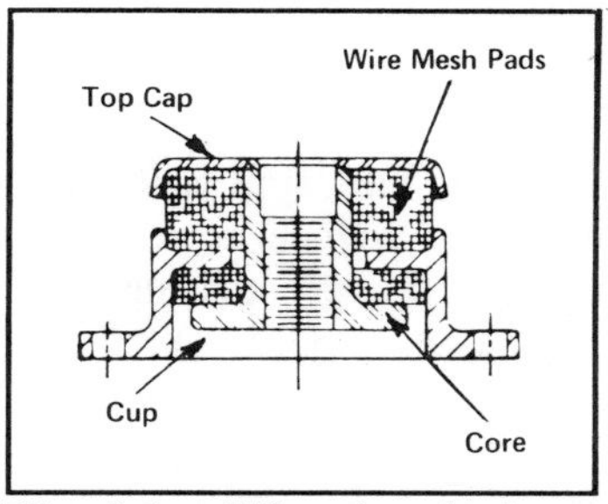

Fig 6-6 - Vibration isolator with steel mesh elements

Pneumatic Vibration Isolators

Pneumatic vibration isolators are air filled reinforced rubber bellows with mounting plates on top and bottom. Isolators such as these can provide very low natural resonant frequencies with small static deflections. With a steel spring type isolator, a 1 Hz natural frequency requires a 10 inch static deflection. A steel spring capable of deflecting 10 inches would have to be about 2 feet long, would be difficult to install, and would present lateral stability problems. There are several types of pneumatic vibration isolators in common use. They include the conventional air spring mount, pneumatic-elastomeric mount, and the active pneumatic isolator.

This type of isolator is basically a pressurized reinforced elastomeric bladder or sleeve affixed between metal end caps. In this design almost all the load is supported by the column of air and not by the sidewalls whose basic function it is to contain the air. With this type of mount, the rubber and the air provide support and resilience, and prevent susceptibility to drift and compression set. The mount will continue to support the equipment weight and isolate even with no air pressure. By proper sizing and distribution of the rubber construction, a low profile, very stable, and low natural-frequency isolator mount can be obtained with built-in shock overload protection, built-in damping, and without the need for external lateral stability provisions (Figure 6-7).

Active Pneumatic Isolation Systems

Active systems reduce natural frequency, isolate "micro-g" vibrations, and automatically maintain loaded height accuracies by using height sensing valves with a continuous air supply connected to special servo-controlled air mounts.

Inertia Bases

A vibration isolation system sometimes consists of an inertial mass supported by vibration isolators. Inertia base frames are often designed and engineered to receive poured concrete. They are intended for use with mechanical equipment. Typically requiring a reinforced concrete inertia base, in turn supported by vibration isolators, they become part of the noise and vibration isolation of the equipment.

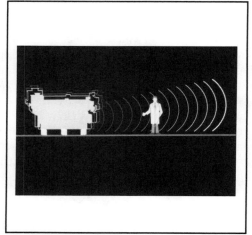

Fig. 6-7 - Typical vibration isolators

Inertia bases reduce vibration amplitude, provide for attachment of vibration isolators, prevent differential movement between driving and driven members, reduce rocking by lowering equipment center of gravity, reduce motion of equipment during start-up and shutdown, act to reduce reaction movement due to operating loads on equipment, and act to reduce the system natural frequency by increasing the mass supported by the vibration isolators.

In some applications, flexible couplings are required as part of the vibration isolation system. Some of the most common vibration sources in industrial facilities are compressors and pumps. Simple vibration isolation of these items from the floor generally is of only limited benefit. This is due to the high amplitude of vibrations which are transmitted along the connecting piping to many other areas of the plant. In addition, mounting brackets for the piping will frequently act to short-circuit the equipment isolators so as to make them almost totally ineffective. Consequently, it is usually necessary to support the piping on, or hung by, vibration isolators. Of further benefit is the prevention of vibration coupling to the piping in the first place. For this purpose flexible piping connectors are available.

Flexible couplings such as these act as vibration breaks in the piping system and ease the problems of pump to pipe alignment when the pump must be vibration isolated from its support structure.

SUMMARY

Vibration isolation materials are generally springs and resilient mounts that are inserted between the driving object and the driven object. Materials may be elastomers, elastomeric foam, cork, felt, fiberglass boards and steel springs, pads or hangers. Design of the correct isolation mount can be predicted by using the formulas developed for specific materials or systems. A key element to the success of the mount is to be sure they are installed per the manufacturers instructions. A spring mount that is bolted down tightly to prevent the machine from vibrating freely from the support will not be effective.

****

Chapter 7 - SYSTEMS FOR NOISE CONTROL

SYSTEM TYPES

Systems for noise and vibration control are finished products or components generally designed for specific purposes. These can be special custom-made items or off-the-shelf stock. Catalog listings are generally laboratory or field tested performance ratings. Most of these products combine sound absorption, sound barrier, vibration damping and isolation into a single item. The degree to which each is incorporated depends on the use for which a specific product is intended. Products are classified into one of four groupings, based on the principal function for which the product is designated. These four groupings are:

- Sound Absorptive Systems
- Sound Barrier Systems
- Silencers
- Vibration/Shock Control Systems

Sound absorptive Systems are designed primarily for absorbing sound that is incident upon their facing surfaces. Such systems may or may not be good sound barriers. For example, ceilings are generally designed for sound absorption but sometimes it is desirable to have a ceiling be a barrier as well and so some ceiling systems have been designed to do both.

Sound barrier systems are designed to prevent the transmission of noise from one space to another space. Also, because of the reverberant buildup of sound in enclosed areas, these systems may be provided with sound absorptive treatment to assist in reducing the resultant transmitted noise. To improve the sound barrier performance in the region of the coincidence dip, many sound barrier systems incorporate vibration damping treatment and/or vibration isolation mountings. A well-designed total machine enclosure, which must have high noise reduction capability, will usually incorporate all these features.

Silencers are devices used in piping or ducted systems to reduce the amount of sound that is transmitted from one section of the system to the next section, or to the atmosphere. These devices are designed to perform noise reduction while at the same time permitting the passage of air or fluid that is flowing in the system. The mechanism for noise control include absorption, barriers, mismatch, or the new technology called "active noise control."

Vibration/shock control systems are designed to prevent the transmission of vibration or shock from the driving member to the driven member. Such a system does not utilize sound absorption or sound barrier properties, but damping is frequently included.

SOUND ABSORPTIVE SYSTEMS

Systems for sound absorption belong to one of two basic categories: free systems and structural systems. Free sound absorbing systems are sound absorbing units that are not part of the structural system, are generally individually supported, and usually can be moved easily. Free systems include such items as hanging unit absorbers or open plan landscape screens. Structural sound absorption systems are incorporated into the construction of the building and form a part of the overall structure. Such systems include absorptive roof decks, ceilings, and curtain walls. The purpose of all sound absorptive systems is to reduce the noise buildup within a space by absorbing the sounds before or during the reflection from the space boundaries. An ideal sound absorptive system is exhibited by the open sky, since all sounds directed at the sky are not reflected back. The result is a reduction of noise levels and echoes making the space acoustically more desirable.

A methodology for predicting the reverberation time and noise reduction achieved by adding sound absorptive materials and systems to a room is presented in Appendix 3. With a knowledge of the sound absorption coefficients of all the room surfaces, including furniture, panels, baffles, ceilings, wall treatments, floor coverings and people, and with knowledge of the room dimensions, one can predict with considerable accuracy the reverberation time at individual frequencies. This data will also predict the degree of noise reduction that can be expected by adding absorbing materials and systems. Data for a range of typical materials may be found in Appendix 4 and in manufacturers technical data.

Ceilings

Probably the most commonly used sound absorptive system is the ceiling system. There are many types of acoustical ceilings, ranging from the attractive tiles seen in homes and offices to the thicker, sturdier panels that can be used in an industrial atmosphere. The absorption ability of modern acoustical ceilings from an NRC of about 0.30 to over 1.00 (Figure 7-1).

From a sampling of the tests performed at acoustical testing laboratories, the most common NRC value is about 0.55 to 0.70. This sampling includes ceilings made of wood fiber, glass fiber, and other mineral fibers. It also includes the full range of densities and thickness, that are common to ceilings. The most efficient absorbers are light density glass or mineral fiber boards made by the dry process. NRCs as high as 1.00 are achievable with 1-1/2" thick product in the 4-6 lb. density range. Most conventional wood and mineral ceiling tiles made by a wet process with densities in the 10-20 lb. range have NRC's from .50 to .60.

Note that ceilings are usually tested in accordance with ASTM procedure C-423 on an E-405 mounting having a 16" plenum behind the ceiling material (Figure 2-6 for mounting types) The effect of this mounting is to increase the absorption in the lower frequency range over that which would be obtained on a Type A mounting with the material mounted directly to the surface.

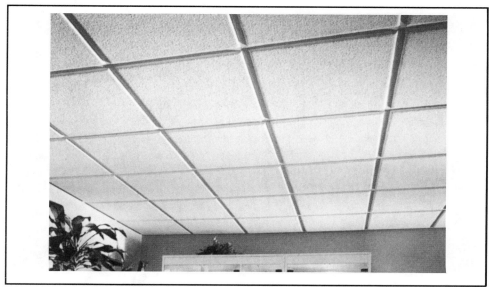

Figure 7-1 - Typical suspended ceiling system.

It is therefore imperative that test data be compared on material with the same mounting. Likewise, the full set of frequency data should be reviewed. Choose the products that perform best in the frequency spectrum predominant in the space where it will be utilized. For example, to remove high frequency noise, select a product that has superior sound absorption coefficients at higher bandwidths. Conversely, to reduce low frequency noise or rumble, focus on the sound absorption coefficients at the lower end of the frequency spectrum. The NRC, while it is a convenient single number rating, is only an average and may not provide sufficient information to select the product for your particular situation. It is intended primarily for speech noise and will be misleading for most industrial noise control applications.

Ceiling systems are comprised of the ceiling board, support grid, HVAC outlets, lights, and other like elements. While most evaluations are made using ceiling board absorption data the other elements of the system could have a detrimental effect on predictive results. For example, some ceiling systems contain up to 50% light fixtures with highly sound reflective lens. Clearly, calculations made on this system must include the absorption of the fixture lens and the ceiling tile as a percent of the total ceiling area. While grid and other ceiling elements are usually of insignificant quantity compared to the ceiling surface area as a whole, they can have an affect. Coffered or vaulted ceiling systems present a particular concern. If possible, sound absorption values should be obtained on the system as a whole. Since there is added surface area and therefore more absorption potential, these systems tend to provide greater Sabines of Absorption in the room. However, there are subtleties that occur at various frequencies that may adversely affect predicted values.

66 NOISE CONTROL MANUAL

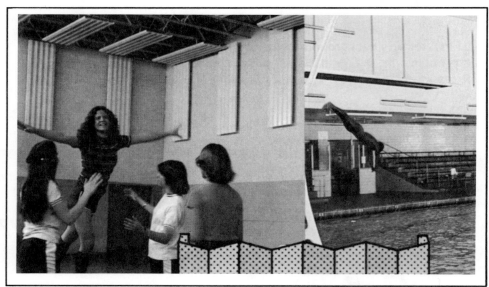

Figure 7-2 - Perforated metal panels with absorbing backing for hard use areas.

Roof Decks and Exposed Floor Systems

The exposed underside or ceiling side of roof and floor decks may be designed to have a sound absorptive surface. Sound absorption is achieved by rendering the exposed surface sound absorptive (Figure 7-2). In some systems, sound is absorbed by placing sound absorbing pads in the interstitial space behind a perforated steel deck system. The ceiling face is perforated to allow sound to reach the absorbing media (see chapter 2 for more information). Spray on fireproofing type materials of a soft, fluffy, or porous nature. Add-on ceiling panels or systems are also common. Recent "hi-tech" architectural design has caused the underside of roof decks to be directly exposed in relatively large office rooms, churches, schools, factories, etc. The additional sound absorption provided by these special acoustical designs helps reduce the reverberation time of the rooms. Test mountings are usually specified as Type A (mountings are described in Appendix 4 - Acoustical Data).

Wall Treatments

Facings in the form of panels, boards, etc., can be mounted on the walls to increase the sound absorption and thus improve the acoustic characteristics of the room. The facings are made from a variety of materials and are available in coverings with pleasing colors and surface textures (Figure 7-3). Ranging from thin films, open weave cloth, wire mesh and perforated metal, the facings can be mounted on a wall in a variety of ways. Backing materials usually consist of a highly absorptive material such as glass fiber. Sound absorption performance is usually a function of the thickness of the sound absorbing material especially for the lower frequencies.

Spacing the wall treatment away from the wall provides an effective increase in thickness and a corresponding increase in absorption at many frequencies. In addition to full wall covering, decorative absorbers are also available.

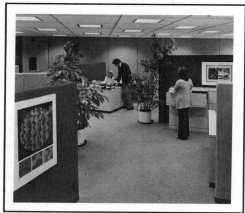

Figure 7-3 - Decorative sound absorbing wall panels.

Test data for comparisons should be specified for a Type A Mounting (i.e. direct to hard surface) unless details indicate otherwise. Note that covering materials will have a significant effect on performance. Unless the covering has 20-30 percent open area and will not impede the flow of sound to the base board, it is imperative that test data be compared on the finished and faced product. Where specific angles of incident sound are likely, a special analysis of the material is warranted. While no formalized procedures are available, an adaptation of the open office test procedure is appropriate (see chapter 8).

Part-or Full-Height Space Dividers or Partitions

Part-or full-height partitions may be used to temporarily or permanently divide a room. In a factory or school, they may be mobile to screen off a particularly noisy area. In an open plan office these dividers may be called moveable screens, acoustical screens, systems furniture, or part-high demountable partitions (Figure 7-3). (For a more detailed description of open office acoustics, see chapter 9.) These systems are generally available with highly sound absorbent facings to reduce the possibility of speech sounds reflecting from a surface into an adjoining work space. Note that their use for absorption within the space to reduce reverberation is usually not required since other absorption from the ceilings and carpets will usually suffice. Part-high barriers should also have a sound barrier septum to block direct sound travel from a source to a receiver location. The presence of a septum could have a significant adverse impact on the sound absorption characteristics of some systems. In closed offices the full-height walls may have permanently affixed sound absorptive faces.

When used strictly for sound absorptive purposes, that is, to reduce reverberation, these units should be evaluated with test data on a Type A mounting. Free standing screens may be tested as a single unit. Note however, that in 1984, ASTM removed the free standing screen mounting from E-996 in 1984 to avoid misuse. These units are more appropriately tested to determine their speech privacy characteristics. See chapter 3 for more information on the design of partitions for their sound barrier characteristics. A whole series of specific procedures have been developed to evaluate part-high space dividers in the open plan office. See chapter 9 for additional information.

Functional Absorbers

Sound absorption inside a room can be increased by adding unit absorbers specially designed for this purpose (Figure 7-4). These units are easily installed, usually on hooks, hangers or stretched wire, and are available in various forms such as baffles, banners, beams, blankets, and freestanding room dividers etc. They may be shaped as flat panels, drums, cylinders, triads, or boxes. Typical installations include multipurpose rooms such as gymnasiums, auditoriums, and natatoriums, where noise buildup causes speech interference. The units are best installed near the noise source. In a large space they should be spread uniformly about the room. Most installations are ceiling suspensions or wall mounting, or both.

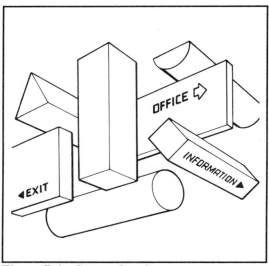

Figure 7-4 - Space absorbers.

The amount of sound energy absorbed by a particular unit absorber is proportional to the area exposed to the incident sound energy. For this reason many absorbers are suspended from ceilings using wires to expose all surfaces to the sound field.

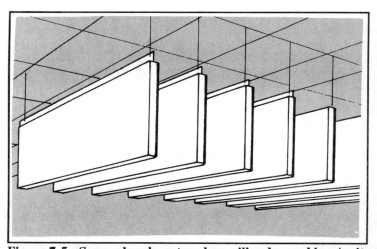

Figure 7-5 - Space absorbers too close will reduce sabines/unit.

Sound absorption data for these units are usually expressed as Sabines/unit at specific frequency bandwidths. Sound absorption coefficients and NRC are not determined since the absorption coefficients are dependent on the number and spacing of the absorbers. As the number of units is increased and the space between them decreases, the total absorption increases but the absorption per unit decreases (Figure 7-5). Reported data (Sabines per unit) for a single unit will therefore be higher than average data for a stacked array. Since discrete frequency noises may be identified in most industrial noise conditions, selection of the units should provide optimum absorption in the same frequency band where the discrete frequency occurs. For broadband noise such as speech, an average absorption from 150 - 4000 Hz may suffice.

SOUND BARRIER SYSTEMS

Sound barriers take a number of forms. They may be a simple wall or floor/ceiling between offices or living units, an enclosure around a noise producer such as a machine or pipe, or a complex building system where interfaces between building elements and the penetrations for pipes and ducts become part of the noise barrier system. Noise "leaks" and "flanking paths" are the nemesis of nearly every well designed sound barrier system as sound, like water and air, will seek the path of least resistance. When selecting a sound barrier system one should always consider the practicality of installing the barrier to eliminate leaks or flanking. Otherwise, the barrier will not provide the real world sound attenuation that it was designed to achieve.

Ceilings

While ceilings are usually considered absorption systems, the open plenum above the ceiling provides a good transmission path for noise to propagate between rooms. For this reason, ceilings should also be a sound barrier. The sound barrier characteristics of a ceiling system are evaluated in a facility that approximates a typical commercial office building. Called AMA I-II (an ASTM version is underway), the test facility is a source/receiver room with a common ceiling (Figure 7-6). The main sound path is via the ceiling plenum. Test results

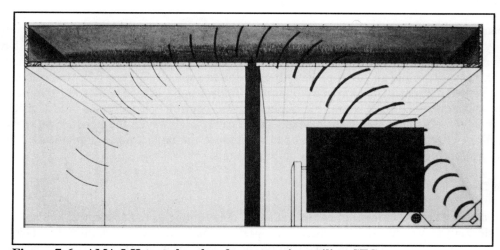

Figure 7-6 - AMA I-II test chamber for measuring ceiling STC.

are in terms of the sound attenuation with a single number rating system called the Sound Transmission Class (STC). Note that the sound signal passes through the ceiling system twice to reach the receiver location. To evaluate noises generated within the ceiling plenum, special test techniques evaluating the single pass transmission loss should be utilized.

Ceiling STC values of 30 to 50 are generally achievable with commercially available ceiling systems. These STC values should match those for the interfacing building elements so that the ceiling system is not a "flanking path." When evaluating the test data, the method used for installing the ceiling system should be carefully noted. The terms "interrupted" or "continuous" mean the ceiling is broken or continuous over the wall. Sound is more likely to be transmitted via the ceiling itself in a continuous installation. Note also the type of ceiling suspension system and how snugly the panels are installed since the most likely degradation of the ceiling board occurs at joint leaks.

Floor/Ceiling Systems (Airborne and Impact)

Airborne sound transmission loss may be evaluated using ASTM test procedure E-90 or one of several equivalent field procedures. The path between the source and receiving location is isolated to the floor/ceiling system. Sound attenuation at frequencies between 125 Hz and 4000 Hz is reported along with the Sound Transmission Class (STC). Floor/ceiling systems typically become better airborne sound barriers as they become heavier. However, considerable research has revealed that lightweight systems incorporating a resilient mounting of one face, typically the ceiling side, with a highly sound absorptive core material, such as mineral building insulation, will provide STCs from 35 to 60. As in all barrier systems, "leaks" and "flanking" must be carefully controlled to achieve the full benefit of the system transmission loss design. See Appendix 4 for a list of STC values for typical floor/ceiling assemblies.

Impact noise isolation from people walking and/or other impacts is a key concern for multi-family residences such as apartments, hotels and condominiums. Several special tests have been developed to evaluate the impact noise. An ASTM and ISO version utilizes a standard tapping machine while an AMA procedure utilizes a live walker (Figure 7-7). In both cases, it is readily apparent that improved isolation of impact noise can be achieved by using the same techniques described above for airborne noise control (i.e. increased mass, resilient attachments and sound absorbent blankets in the cavity). However, the flooring will have a significant effect. Clearly, a carpet and pad will reduce the impact noise dramatically. Soft or foam flooring materials are definite improvements.

Roof Decks

Roof decking can be thought of as the industrial counterpart to the absorptive ceiling. But roof decking also provides sound barrier properties, since there will generally be a layer of tar, tar paper, and gravel or other material on the outside for weather purposes. Some styles of roof deck systems come in different thickness, and provide a different degree of sound

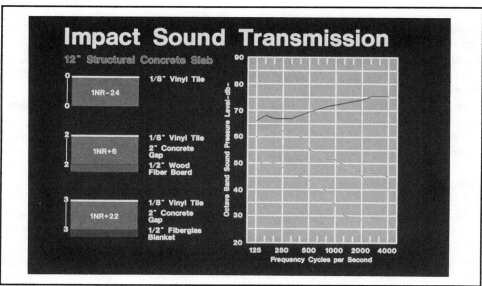

Figure 7-7 - Impact noise rating examples.

absorption and sound attenuation depending on the thickness and on the type of buildup roof backing used. A roof deck may be evaluated for its airborne sound transmission loss in the same manner as the floor/ceiling system described above. STC values and system techniques for improving them will also be similar.

Partition Systems

Interior, exterior and party wall systems have been extensively researched over the years to improve their sound transmission loss characteristics and efficiency. In early testing, barriers were improved by increasing the mass. The mass law implied that for each doubling of the weight per square foot, one could improve the sound transmission loss by 6 dB. Since construction practices would not accommodate the added weight and cost, many partition systems evolved utilizing separate studded walls (i.e. staggered studs), sound deadening board (i.e. a wood fiber sheet underlayer), resilient furring channels to acoustically isolate or decouple one or both wall faces, and the addition of sound absorbing insulation blankets in the core. These principals were extended to the drywall steel stud systems which provide an inherently resilient mount.

The preferred method for evaluating the sound transmission loss of a partition system is ASTM E-90 or its several variations for field analysis (see chapter 2). AMA I-II is a similar method (Figure 7-6). The test specimen is mounted between an isolated source and a receiving room. Sound transmission loss, the difference between the sound level in the source room and in the receiving room with a normalization factor for room absorption, is measured at test frequencies between 125 and 5000 Hz. The Sound Transmission Class (STC) is then calculated. STC values of 20 to 60 are achieved with commercially available systems. Note that the test data generally eliminates sound leaks or flanking paths. The test report must outline all construction processes and techniques that could affect the sound transmission characteristics of that system. Any deviation from the system description may degrade tested performance. In fact, field performance generally does not measure up to laboratory performance. The reasons are numerous and beyond the scope of this text. To assure that the installed system achieves sound transmission loss capabilities, many specifiers require compliance with ASTM E-497, Standard Practice for Installing Sound-isolating Gypsum Board Partitions.

Demountable Partition Systems

Designed primarily for interior partitions in commercial office buildings, demountable partitions come in many varieties, from prefabricated panels to a series of assembled components. Facings may be steel clad, gypsum board or the popular textured vinyl. Sound transmission loss performance, design, and testing are essentially the same as for fixed wall systems. Systems with STC values of 30 to 60 are commercially available. Since these systems will be installed and removed several times during their useful life they are particularly vulnerable to sound leaks. Instead of caulking materials to seal cracks, compressible foams and weather seal techniques are typically used at panel joints and interfaces. It is recommended that the user retest the system after installation or reconfiguration to assure that the seals are maintained in the original condition.

Sound absorbing face panels on demountable partitions are also growing in popularity. Designers want partitions with high STC ratings and high NRC values in a system that will provide 1 and 2 hour fire ratings, is structurally sound, costs little, is easily demounted for relocation, and has a monolithic appearance. Just such a partition system has been invented by D. A. Harris (Figure 7-8). All these performance requirements place an extra demand on maintaining acoustical integrity and the special care of the installer.

Special criteria for interfaces with the ceiling system may require unique solutions. For example, a sound absorbing lined interface cap was developed for a large government project where the partition never touched the ceiling. By using an acoustically lined cap that provided structural stability, STC values of up to 45 were maintained with a 1/2" air gap along the ceiling/partition interface.

Operable Partitions

In addition to rigid, permanent, and demountable walls, it is desirable to be able to move, fold or relocate partitions frequently. Operable partitions, or room dividers, are easily folded or extended by anyone who wants to divide the room on a temporary basis. Typically suspended from an overhead track, many ride on rolling bearings for ease of operation. Many styles and configurations are available. Their use in hotels, convention centers and schools is widespread. Sound transmission loss values of STC 20 to 50 are commercially available. To ensure that the acoustical integrity of the system is maintained over its life span, many specifiers require compliance with ASTM E-557, Standard Practice for Architectural Application and Installation of Operable Partitions.

Moveable Wall Systems

Acoustical moveable wall systems have been used for many years to acoustically divide public and private meeting areas so that events can occur on either side of the moveable wall without concern for privacy or interference from intruding noise.

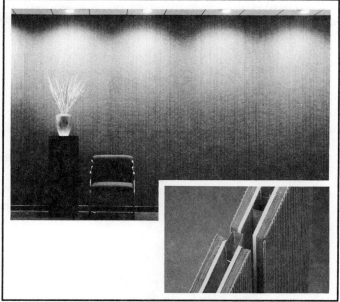

Figure 7-8 - Acoustical Partition (Inventor; D. A. Harris)

Architects and engineers have been faced with some unusual design problems caused by the very tall floor/ceiling heights, some up to 30 or 40 feet and spans from 200 to 300 feet.

These requirements typically occur in convention centers and as a result, need product features in addition to sound isolation. Live load deflections of up to 6 inches while maintaining tight acoustical seals are a significant challenge. In addition, the systems sometimes require pressure relief silencers to equalize air pressure buildup on either side of the wall.

Sound Control Panels

A variety of acoustical building block panel components are available to solve many industrial and architectural noise problems (see chapter 9 for office screens). These panels typically have a back side of a heavy sound barrier material with a perforated metal inner facing. Between these two layers is a porous sound absorptive material. The perforated facing permits sound to enter the porous absorptive material to prevent reverberant sound buildup, while the heavy backing provides the sound transmission loss or barrier property.

Available in panel thicknesses of 2" to 12", the thicker panels have better sound absorption and barrier properties. By adding additional layers of lead or gypsum board, the STC may be upgraded. All of the panels are designed with some form of interlocking channel on all four edges to insure a tight seal when multiple units are used to construct a larger surface or an enclosure. Mounted on wheels, they become temporary sound barriers particularly suited for industrial applications. Other uses include lagging for large fans and ductwork.

Enclosures

The use of a single sound control panel will usually not result in much sound reduction due to diffraction and reflection of sound around the ends, edges and top. Consequently, a total, or almost total, enclosure is necessary (Figures 7-9 and 7-10).

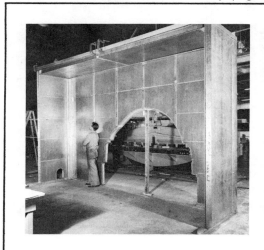

Figure 7-9 - Enclosure designed to block noise generated by a large power plant turbine.

An enclosure is defined as a covering that attenuates the sound emanating from the inside, as opposed to a "quiet room" where the unwanted noise originates outside. It is difficult to provide meaningful transmission loss information about enclosures because the performance depends on how the enclosure fits around a particular machine. The size of openings that are required to satisfy machine operational requirements and other penetrations also affect sound attenuation. For existing machinery, total or partial enclosures are often the most economical solutions to the noise control problem. Such enclosures are frequently custom designed to suit particular requirements.

Caution; an item that generates noise probably also generates heat. A sound enclosure is also a heat enclosure with a corresponding increase in temperature inside. For this reason, many enclosures are fitted with ventilating air systems with appropriate sound treated air passages (see lined ducts for design information).

Quiet Rooms

Personnel enclosures placed on the factory floor containing equipment controls are an effective means of satisfying noise control regulations (Figure 7-11). Designed to block intruding noise from the outside and to provide a quiet haven, these enclosures also require other environmental controls including temperature and air quality controls. These rooms may provide a variety of functions. They may provide a quiet haven for a worker in a noisy factory, a suitable space for audiometric testing, a place for music recording, or a booth for telephone calls. With construction similar to the acoustical panels described above, moderate to excellent noise reductions are available in commercially produced units. Testing of these units has been performed in several ways. ASTM Committee E33 is presently preparing a

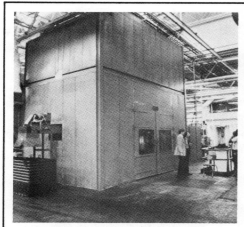 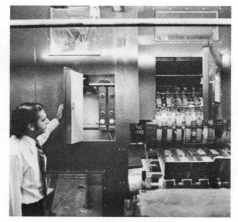

Large punch press is entirely enclosed in acoustical structure.   *Enclosure for printing press includes acoustically effective access doors and windows.*

Figure 7-10 - Enclosure Examples

uniform procedure. Noise reduction is a function of panel design for sound transmission loss and proper sealing of sound leaks.

Pre-assembled Structures and Modules

A wide variety of pre-assembled acoustical structures have been furnished to meet OSHA, EPA and other industry criteria. Pre-assembled structures such as in-plant offices have been shipped completely assembled and ready for immediate use.

Structures of this type ensure factory built quality, reduce downtime at the site, and keep field labor costs at a minimum. These pre-assembled structures are constructed from a great variety of panel types and designs and may include silencers, acoustical windows and single/double leaf doors. Most are equipped to be picked up by a fork-lift or crane and typical weights may be on the order of 1 to 3 tons.

Doors

A significant noise path in any barrier is an access door. Door manufacturers have done considerable research in recent years to assess the degree of sound transmission through a noise barrier due to the door, frame and the interfacing elements. ASTM E1408 procedure has been written to identify the test procedure for doors and their operation for sound transmission loss. For low sound rated constructions, the typical hollow core door may be upgraded to its potential sound rating of 20 to 25 STC by installing superior sound gaskets and drop closures. Similar to weather seals, the gaskets reduce the sound leaks around the door perimeter. Solid core doors are generally better barriers and will require a better perimeter seal to achieve their sound transmission loss potential. Also, double doors are an obvious improvement. A broad range of industrial doors, usually metal clad, are available in the market place. Many have been specially designed to achieve STC values from 40 to 60 (Figure 7-12). Special seals and latch devices ensure that these doors are operable, and yet will maintain their sound transmission loss potential. To ensure that the doors are functioning to their full potential, field analysis of the sound attenuation of the entire operating door assembly is recommended.

Windows

Apertures for viewing through a noise barrier should have sound transmission loss characteristics similar to the barrier that supports them. Both the glazing and the frame are potential sound leaks. A single pane of 1/4" laminated glass fully sealed in place can achieve an STC of 34. Operable windows will allow sound leakage. For example, a wood double hung window used in residences may have an STC 28 when sealed, 26 when locked and 22 when unlocked. An aluminum operable casement will range from 31 STC when sealed to 17 when unlocked.

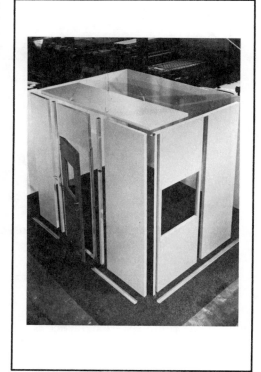

Figure 7-11 - Quiet room or personnel enclosure

For industrial applications, glazing manufacturers have developed special laminated glass and double or triple glazing to improve STC values as high as 50 STC (Figure 7-13). Sound leakage at the frame and interface with the supporting barrier are key factors in maintaining the acoustical integrity of the window systems. Laboratory procedures similar to doors are contained in ASTM E-90. Field analysis per ASTM procedure E966 is recommended to measure the transmission loss of building facades. ASTM E1332 identifies a single number rating called the Outdoor-Indoor Transmission Class (OITC).

Curtains

Sound barrier curtains typically utilize loaded vinyl materials. This material offers flexibility, and strength when reinforced with fiberglass webbing, and the high mass offers good sound barrier properties. The flexibility and natural damping reduce the effect of the coincidence

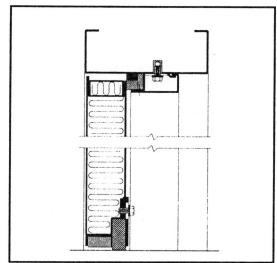

Figure 7-12 - Cross section of a door with a high STC. Automatic drop seals and compressed gaskets are vital.

dip so they behave similar to their theoretical mass law curve.

When mounted with proper hangers and rails, these curtains can be operated like regular draperies so that the area enclosed by the curtain is easily accessible. Operable partitions between rooms and machinery enclosures are common uses for these curtains. They are also available with an absorptive inner facing which can be covered with a thin film for protection.

In many industrial noise control applications, it is not necessary to have 40 to 50 STC reductions in sound level. A partial enclosure may be more than adequate. It should be noted, however, that most of the curtains were tested free hanging in a test opening with their edges sealed to the sides of the opening using a dense flexible mastic. In industrial applications, the sides of the curtains are usually not sealed, with only an overlap for a seal. The result will be a decline in tested values.

Pipe Lagging

Pipe lagging treatment generally consists of a layer of porous sound absorptive material covered by a layer of heavy barrier material (Figure 7-14). The porous material acts both to absorb sound and to provide a vibration isolation or decoupling element to effectively float the barrier away from the piping. Frequently, ease of application, fire resistance, and thermal properties are the determining criteria when selecting a pipe lagging.

Common materials for pipe lagging are elastomeric foams, fiberglass, and mineral wool for the absorptive and decoupling layer. Note that selection must take into consideration the operating temperatures of the materials in the pipes. Since the materials are good thermal insulators, operating temperatures of the pipe will equal the temperatures of the liquid itself. Materials for the outer, or barrier, layer include heavy mastics, loaded vinyl, metallic foils, lead and an array of composite materials. Surface shapes may be smooth, molded or ribbed.

Noise reduction performance should be designed to be optimum for the frequency of sounds that predominate under maximum flow conditions. Since it is likely that the problem sounds will be in a narrow band of frequency, designs should provide optimum attenuation for the offending sounds. Due to the nature of pipe lagging, with complex curved shapes and direct contact between the lagging and pipes, there are important differences between how a material will behave in actual applications and in laboratory analysis. Standard ASTM E-90 transmission loss data will not provide an accurate prediction of the sound attenuation achieved in practice. Consequently, it is recommended that field analysis be conducted on significant projects. A simple measurement of the noise without treatment will identify the intensity and frequency peaks. Comparison tests after application of pipe lagging will reveal the attenuation achieved by the damping, absorption, and barrier characteristics of the lagging. It will also identify sound leaks.

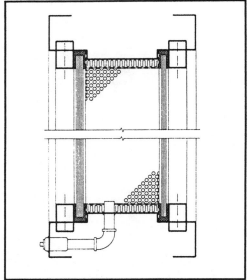

Figure 7-13 - Cross Section of a high STC window unit. Note sound absorbing material at perimeter of frame and tight seals.

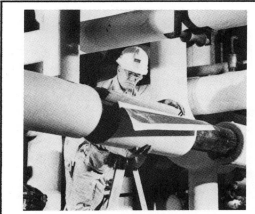

Pipe coverings muffle noisy piping systems. They are also effective unit sound absorbers.

Figure 14 - Pipe lagging

Air Duct Systems

A wide array of sound attenuation devices are available to attenuate the sound that travels down the inside of a tube or air distribution system. The most common treatment is to line the inside of the duct with sound absorbing material such as fiber glass board (Figure 7-15). With the current concern for fibers in the air, the resin content of the material and its ability to hold the fibers in place or, coverings containing the fibers, should be addressed. Polyolyphine films that are tough and under 1 mill thick have been used effectively without negating the sound absorbing properties of the absorber. Open cell foams also perform well in duct attenuation. Devices called "duct attenuators" specially designed to be very efficient absorbers are widely used in high air flow locations or where the noise source is too close to the receiver location to use other means. Additional information on the function of air duct attenuators may be found in chapter 5, with performance information in Appendix 4. Active duct systems are discussed fully in Chapter 5.

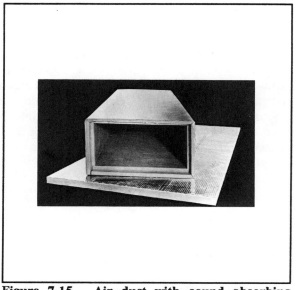

Figure 7-15 - Air duct with sound absorbing interior lining attenuates sound transmission down the duct.

SUMMARY

Systems for noise control may encompass one or more of the four basic groupings including sound absorption, sound barriers, silencers and vibration/shock control. Absorptive systems include ceilings, exposed floor systems, wall treatments and functional absorbers. Barrier systems may be part or full height space dividers or partitions, floor/ceilings, enclosures, and quiet rooms. Doors, windows, HVAC ducts, interfaces and all penetrations have a significant impact on the sound barrier characteristics of the complete assembly. Care should be taken to assure that the systems are installed in accordance with accepted industry practice or the manufacturers recommendations.

****

Chapter 8 - OFFICE ACOUSTICS

OFFICE ACOUSTICS ARE CHANGING

Dramatic changes in the office work force in recent years due to takeovers, downsizing, and technological innovation have caused a startling redefinition of user needs. As a result, the flexibility required of the office environment has been strained to the limit. No environmental element has been spared this reevaluation, including acoustics. Adding to the complex and demanding environment, designers are now mixing closed and open office designs. Providing optimum speech privacy requires an interdisciplinary effort and a holistic approach, emphasizing the need to integrate acoustical design with lighting, HVAC, fire safety, and power and signal distribution for a safe, efficient and cost-effective office environment. Heralded as the wave of the future over 10 years ago, a design methodology utilizing a systems concept is imperative in today's demand for optimum speech privacy.

Through the decade of the 70s, innovations such as the "open office" and "Bureaulaundshaft" (landscape office) swept through the design field, making it an exciting time to be designing offices. The 80s brought new research and a plethora of new products designed specifically to meet the stringent demands for speech privacy in the open plan. Acoustical jargon such as Background Masking, Speech Privacy Noise Isolation Class (NIC'), Speech Privacy Potential (SPP), and a host of others permeated manufacturers literature, design publications and facilities management journals.

The late 80s brought a new design trend to mix open and closed offices and new acoustical consensus standards for testing and specifications. Just when many were beginning to grasp the technology of open office acoustics, including the massive use of highly efficient sound absorbing materials and electronic masking sound, both material criteria and terminology changed. *After 15 years of discussion, we now have a set of industry consensus standards on office acoustics.* Issued by the American Society of Testing and Materials (ASTM), Committee E-33 on Environmental Acoustics, they are based on the same technology used in the well known PBS C.1 and C.2 standards. We now have new rating systems such as Articulation Class (AC) and Articulation Index (AI). These new procedures require materials and systems be retested. To meet the demands of the closed/open office layouts, new materials and systems are also required.

CHALLENGE OF THE 90s

The challenge we face in the 90s is to design office environments for comfort, convenience and efficiency. Only with an optimum acoustical environment can management achieve the increased productivity they promised. Confirmation of the relationship between acoustics and productivity has been verified by every study of office efficiency. They all state that the human performer must have an optimum acoustical environment to be productive. Achieving this high level of performance requires a comprehensive analysis of user acoustical needs. Translated into acoustical design criteria using the new ASTM procedures, a successful acoustical environment can be achieved provided that there is an exacting application of acoustical systems. A systems solution will bring together experts in design, acoustics, specifications, manufacturing, and from contracting. An implementation plan that leaves out any person responsible for the bottom line is destined to be "an eavesdropper's paradise."

THE SOUND OF SILENCE

To those who spent many years learning the basics of Sound Transmission Loss through a partition or floor/ceiling assembly, you found that higher Sound Transmission Class (STC) ratings meant better acoustical privacy. System designs that provided a good sound barrier were heavy, constructed of limp materials, or utilized resilient supported faces with fibrous blanket cores. These barriers were only as good as laboratory tests indicated when special measures were implemented by the installer to eliminate "flanking paths." Massive use of expensive acoustical sealants carefully applied by the contractor were required. By contrast, sound absorbing materials, rated by their Noise Reduction Class (NRC), were added to an occupied space to reduce the reverberation time or echoing. The more absorption material added to a space, the better one could understand speech. Absorbing materials also lowered the ambient sound level. STC and NRC ratings worked well for their specific application. They still are the appropriate way to select materials and systems for the environment intended (namely multi-family dwellings or closed offices) and to reduce reverberation in commercial spaces.

According to the new ASTM documents, *STC and NRC are inappropriate measurement tools for the open plan office.* The properties measured are not applicable. Why? First, barriers in an open plan rarely, if ever, provide an opportunity to eliminate flanking paths. By definition, they are only part-high and discontinuous, allowing sounds to reflect easily over and around them. Even in an ideal environment, such as the open sky where sounds have nothing to reflect them, open office barriers need not exceed 20 STC. This degree of sound attenuation is easily achieved with a simple sheet of 1/8" hardboard, sheet metal or even layers of foil.

A key design goal of open office barriers is flexibility and the ability to be reconfigured into new office layouts. These barriers will move many times in their life span. Often the barriers will be located in a position where they reflect sounds around another barrier. This is called the flanking position. To avoid flanking, barrier faces must be rendered highly sound absorbent. Using NRC values to evaluate the sound absorbing properties of an open office barrier is insufficient. By design, NRC measures the absorptive characteristics at *all angles* of incident sound. In an open plan office, flanking sounds occur overwhelmingly at angles of incidence between 45 and 60 degrees. Materials that exhibit a high NRC are not always effective absorbers at the desired angles, thereby creating a need for a more specific means to measure the sound absorptive characteristics of open office barriers. The same analysis is applicable to the ceiling in an open office. A prime area of reflected sound, ceilings must be highly absorbent in the 45 to 60 degree angle of incident sound. These are the angles that reflect source sounds to an adjoining work station. While many materials having NRCs greater than 0.90 do provide good speech privacy, there are some that are ineffective at the required angles of reflection. Again NRC is not an effective tool to measure the speech privacy performance of a ceiling.

TEST DEVELOPMENT

From the onset, acousticians recognized the need for a set of test procedures that measured the effectiveness of both materials and the resultant environment to provide speech privacy in the open plan office. Speech is the prime acoustical element in open office acoustics. The ultimate goal is to provide degrees of speech privacy suitable for the user need. The term "normal speech privacy" applies to those situations such as a secretarial station, where minor intrusions are acceptable . "Confidential speech privacy" denotes a work station where the sense of an adjoining conversation is not discernable. Since speech has a substantially different sound spectrum than that measured by NRC and STC, a new procedure was required. When research findings indicated that some materials worked better than others in providing speech privacy, even though they had the same NRC or STC, it became obvious that the old procedures were not measuring the real world. And the third element of speech privacy, masking sound, had no convenient measurement procedure.

It was recognized early on that to achieve any degree of speech privacy between work stations in an open plan, careful control of both the signal distribution and background sounds was required. The environment that provides "confidential privacy" *requires all three elements - ceiling, barriers and background masking sound. It is an "all-or-nothing situation"* (Figure 8-1). Similar to the weak link in the chain concept, all three elements must be optimum to achieve speech privacy. Specifically, the ceiling must absorb reflected sounds almost as effectively as the open sky. Barriers must not leak direct sounds and must have sound absorbing surfaces nearly as effective as the ceiling when in the flanking position. Electronic masking sound must exhibit spatial and temporal uniformity throughout the occupied space and have a spectrum shape that is loud enough to be effective as a mask but not so loud as to be obtrusive. Measurement of background masking sounds requires more than a simple sound level measurement. Even a slight difference in level or spectrum makes the difference between achieving confidential speech privacy and no speech privacy. *The goal in acoustical terms is a "signal to noise ratio" approaching zero.* In that environment even a slight change in either the signal or background will cause a significant listener reaction. Similar to two slightly different white colors on opposite walls, a difference in speech privacy, with a wide signal to noise ratio, is difficult to notice. Place the two paints on the same wall, or provide a signal to noise ratio near zero, and the difference is obvious. Hence, leaving out any one of the elements (screen, ceiling and masking) will make the achievement of speech privacy at any level an impossible task. In fact, using only the absorbing materials without masking will make the situation worse since absorbing materials tend to remove natural masking sounds causing the signal to noise ratio to widen rather than approach zero.

To meet all these exacting needs, the U.S. General Services Administration (GSA) enlisted the support of Geiger and Hamme (G&H) Laboratories to develop appropriate measurement procedures (Figure 8-2) Starting with simple tests on the roof of their laboratory with the open sky as a perfect absorber, and by contrast, conducting tests in a chamber with a highly sound reflective gypsum board ceiling, G&H evolved a whole new technology. For many years the resulting specifications issued by the GSA Public Buildings Service (PBS), known as PBS C.1 and C.2, were the industry norm. They

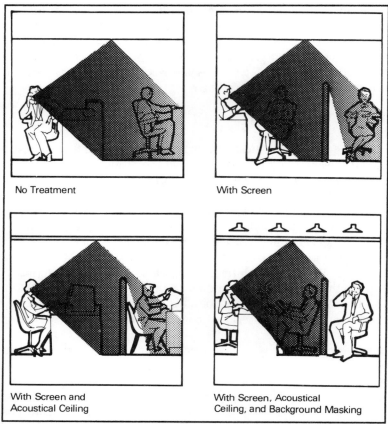

Figure 8-1 - Acoustical treatments for open-plan offices

were used on millions of square feet of government office buildings and private sector projects. These procedures spawned the terms Speech Privacy Potential (SPP) and Speech Privacy Noise Isolation Class (NIC'). Masking sound was rated by the NC_{40} level (NC_{40} being the Noise Criteria Curve of 40).

While technically correct and very effective, a segment of the acoustical community was not fully satisfied with the PBS procedures. For example, the author proposed that the PBS procedures be adopted as ASTM standards over 15 years ago. The ensuing years of discussion at ASTM SubCommittee E-33.02 on Open Plan Acoustics saw many changes in products, systems technology and personalities. For all of these reasons, the new ASTM procedures are different enough from the PBS documents that new rating procedures were required. Being adopted by ASTM makes them truly "industry standards." While some may desire additional detail, these new standards represent a *consensus of the industry* and deserve adoption by all who specify or evaluate open office acoustics. The entire family of documents

Office Acoustics 85

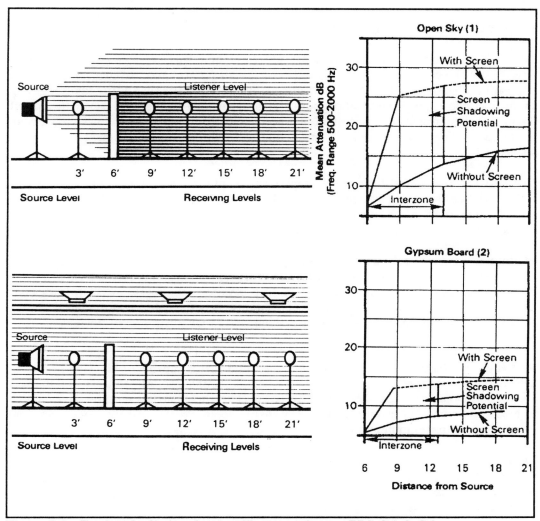

Figure 8-2 - Testing the limits of open office acoustics per PBS C.1 & C.2
Test XL-1LT: (Top) - open sky. Test XL-2LT: (Bottom) gypsumboard ceiling (G&H Labs.)

is not yet adopted, however, the major ones are published and others will follow shortly (See Appendix 3 for description and listing of the standards).

OPEN PLAN PRODUCT AND SYSTEMS SOLUTIONS

Open office acoustical products and system solutions require an integrated systems approach. Specifically, the ceiling, part-high barriers, vertical wall surfaces and masking sound must be compatible acoustically and satisfy all other environmental criteria such as fire safety, lighting, thermal comfort, code compliance, power and signal distribution, and aesthetic appeal. Though they represent only part of all that needs to be considered, the following comments about the ceiling, barriers and masking sound will help assure achievement of optimum speech privacy.

Ceilings: Ceilings comprise the largest single component for reflected sounds in an open plan office. The entire ceiling system, including the grid, board, luminaires and HVAC outlets, must be able to absorb or otherwise deflect source signals between 45 and 60 degrees from normal. 1-1/2" thick glass fiber or light density rock wool boards with porous facings are required. Materials should exhibit an Articulation Class (AC) of 220. Special luminaires that exhibit performance equivalent to the ceiling board are required, or there will be "hot spots." Large cell (4" or larger) parabolic fixtures or "V" lenses with absorbing sides have proven to be successful. HVAC outlets of the standard drop-in variety may negate speech privacy when located in the critical path between two work stations. A better solution is the linear air bar. And not to be overlooked, suspension systems with wide flanges can create a strip of reflections.

Part High Barriers: Barriers must contain a septum that is capable of blocking sounds to a degree compatible with the attenuation from flanking sounds (i.e. AC 220). Typical barriers are 1/8" hardboard or 22 ga. sheet steel. To be effective, these barriers must be large enough to block direct and diffracted sounds. They should be at least 5 feet high, 8 feet wide and have minimum panel joint and floor interface sound leaks (Figure 8-3).

Vertical Surfaces: All vertical surfaces, including furniture panels, walls, square columns, window walls, etc. must have surfaces that exhibit sound absorption similar to the ceiling panels (i.e. AC 220). A common solution is a 1" minimum thickness of glass fiber board with open weave cloth coverings.

Masking: Masking sound systems should be designed to be compatible with the ceiling systems. They must deliver an acceptable sound spectrum in a uniform fashion throughout the occupied space. Specifications call for both temporal and spatial uniformity. Music is not acceptable as masking since it is transient. Electronic systems with dual horn speakers located in the ceiling plenum have been found to be a practical means of providing sound masking (Figures 8-4, 8-5 and 8-6).

CLOSED/OPEN DESIGN DILEMMA:

Mixed closed and open offices that are changed back and forth over time present a special challenge to material and system suppliers. Unfortunately, most material manufacturers have not risen to the challenge; very few solutions are readily available.

Ceilings are particularly bothersome since both sound absorption and sound attenuation are required. In the closed office, the ceiling must block the sound (sound attenuation), while in the open office, ceilings must be nearly perfect absorbers (i.e. the open sky). These two properties are

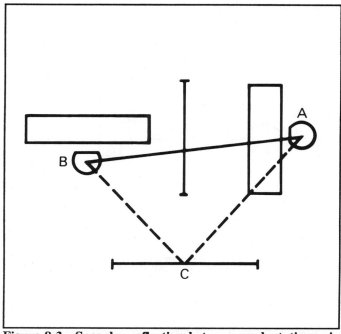

Figure 8-3 - **Specular reflection between work stations via vertical surface C.**

diametrically opposed in most materials. One solution is a ceiling material composed of a sandwich panel with a high sound barrier backing and a highly sound absorbent face (i.e. a gypsum board backer with a thick fiberglass facing covered with open weave fabric). Luminaires pose a special problem since they too must be good absorbers and barriers. The typical fixture that provides acceptable reflective attenuation (note that they are not really absorbers in the true sense) utilize a large cell parabolic design. Parabolic cells must be 4" by 4" or larger to be effective. Small cell parabolic lens react to sound much like an acoustical mirror. Unfortunately, most fixtures have many holes and provide poor sound attenuation. A box that surrounds the back of the fixture like those required in some fire rated systems, seems the only practical solution at the moment. HVAC distribution becomes a real problem as many systems utilize air return light fixtures that allow a direct air path and sound leaks to the common plenum. Returns that can be lined with absorbing material may be required.

Partitions for the closed/open design require demountable systems with sound absorbing faces. While not required (but highly desirable) inside the closed office, walls exposed to the open plan space must be rendered highly sound absorbent and provide an AC in flanking of 220. At least a 1" or thicker glass fiber board with open weave coverings is required. Since most closed/open designs require optimum flexibility, including the ability to change from

88 NOISE CONTROL MANUAL

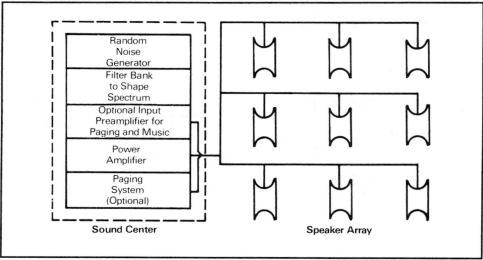

Figure 8-4 - Background Sound Masking System Schematic

closed to open or visa versa overnight, a demountable partition is needed. To meet code and client needs, a 1 hr. fire rating may be required, the system should be able to support systems furniture and provide an STC of 40. Systems that satisfy these criteria are few and very expensive. As a result, some contractors may design a special partition system. The problem is that many designers budget for conventional demountable partitions which typically are one-third the cost. A new partition system that fills this need and provides a monolithic look has been fully developed but not yet marketed. Called MO-DEM, short for monolithic demountable partition, it can provide an STC of 30 to 50, an NRC of 80, an AC of 300 to 550 in the barrier position and up to 220 in the flanking position, 1 hour time design fire rating capability, support hang on systems furniture, space for power and signal distribution at any point, and has an installed cost less than most systems furniture panels.

If a **masking system** is to be deployed in the closed office area, the interior surface of closed offices should have highly absorptive faces. *Masking sound can be used in closed offices.* And in fact, it will enhance the speech privacy of the walls and ceilings dramatically. To be effective, sound levels should be 5 dB_A lower in closed offices than in the open area. A simple loudness adjustment on the speakers will suffice. The use of ceilings with both high absorption and attenuation will require more power than usual. In addition, these systems may not be acceptable for paging or fire management systems since the extra single pass attenuation of the ceiling system may significantly alter the clarity of voice announcements. A system featuring a speaker composed of a "double horn" has been a proven performer in millions of square feet of open plan offices. This system has also been used successfully in closed offices. Previously known as the Sweeny Baffle, this system is now available from Building and Acoustic Design Consultants, (D. A. Harris, Principal - 213 377-9958) To assure masking is acceptable, specify site testing for spatial and temporal (i.e. over time) uniformity per ASTM E1041.

QUIET FLOORS

A new development has occurred in floor systems for small projects and in modular buildings without massive floors. Typical lightweight construction composed of wood or steel joists with a plywood subfloor are notoriously noisy, both to the walker and to the occupant below. A remedy uses subfloor materials with "constrained layer damping." A viscoelastic material, placed at the centroid of the panels, reduces the drum head effect. As a replacement for conventional subfloor materials, the damped panels give the impression of a solid and substantial floor akin to a concrete floor several times heavier and more costly.

HOW TO SPECIFY

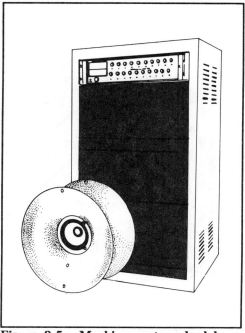

Figure 8-5 - Masking system dual horn speaker and sound center.

The new ASTM specifications provide the basics (see table I at the end of this chapter). However, ASTM documents do not establish acoustical criteria. One must identify user needs and transform them into criteria appropriate for the situation. Unfortunately, this is not as simple as the industry would like. Once it is established whether the user needs normal or confidential privacy and whether there will be open offices, closed offices or a mix of both, documentation does exist to create a set of specifications. With this information in hand an acoustician can create appropriate criteria and identify materials and systems that will achieve the desired performance (an example is given in table II at the end of this chapter). The most vexing problem is finding materials and systems that fit into the aesthetic, building code criteria and budget restrictions established by the space planner or designer. *Caution, do not break up a system solution and leave one of the components out because it is too expensive.* It would be better to ignore acoustics altogether. Remember, speech privacy is an "all-or-nothing situation requiring all three components; highly absorbing ceiling systems, good barriers and wall absorbers, and background masking sound to be effective.

MATERIAL and SYSTEM SELECTION

Specifiers, facilities managers and contractors are already aware of the difficulty in obtaining appropriate acoustical information from manufacturers. Recent takeovers and reorganizations have caused large firms to reduce or eliminate technical staffs, to relegate

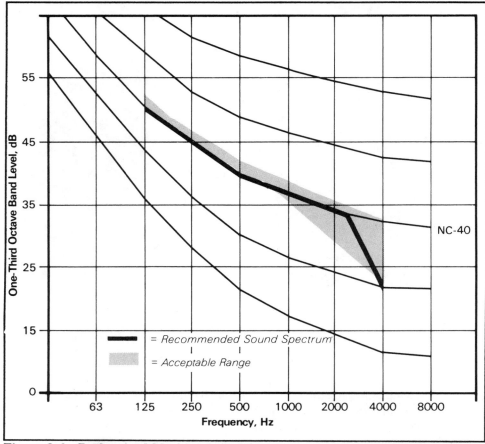

Figure 8-6 - Background Masking Sound Spectrum

sales representatives to the role of order takers and to eliminate specialized product lines. For example, two major ceiling manufacturers have been concentrating on consolidating new found business due to others exiting the industry, rather than providing updated technical information. Several smaller firms that attempted to pick up the slack succumbed to financial woes of their own. As a result, proper acoustical information and specialized products are difficult to acquire. To assure that acoustical success is achieved on your project, the designer and specifier must either become acoustical experts or hire one. To select a consultant either contact the National Council of Acoustical Consultants (NCAC) at (201) 379-1100. Another source is the Noise Control Association (NCA), (213) 377-9958. For more detailed information, the book "Planning and Designing the Office Environment", authored by D. A. Harris, et al, published by Van Nostrand Reinhold, has a full chapter on acoustics. The book emphasizes a "systems approach" to office design. Interfaces between professional disciplines and subsystems such as acoustics, lighting, HVAC, fire safety, and power and signal distribution are carefully addressed to assure the system as a whole provides the desired performance. First published in 1981, the second edition (1991) has been updated and expanded. The ASTM documents provide considerable information, but you will be left on your own to establish criteria. They also assume, the reader is an acoustical expert.

SUMMARY

The importance of implementing a systems approach to optimize office acoustics cannot be overemphasized. There is no single, quick-fix answer. Successful projects are the result of considerable balance and compromise. If done properly, the user will not be aware of the elements that optimize their performance. If done poorly, the red ink of financial failure may indelibly plague the project for its entire useful life. And, retrofit acoustics are notoriously expensive. If good acoustics is important to the success of an office, and we know that it is from all the productivity studies, then proper acoustical planning is a must. To ensure optimum productivity of the human performer, be certain that good acoustics are part of your next project.

****

TABLE I

NEW STANDARDS FOR THE OPEN PLAN OFFICE

The following synopsis describes a family of new standards published by The American Society Testing & Materials (ASTM) Committee E-33 on Environmental Acoustics and Subcommittee E-33.02 on Open Plan Offices. The author is Vice Chairman of Subcommittee E-33.04 (Applications) and participated in preparing many of these documents. Standards with a number designation are, or will be, published in ASTM Volume 04.06. Those listed generically are in the final phases of the consensus standards process.

ASTM E1041 - Guide for Measurement of Masking Sound in Open Offices

Use: Measures variation of masking sound over time and throughout a space, and its correlation to a specified sound spectrum. Can be used as an acceptance or problem solving tool by specifiers.
Result: Spatial and Temporal Uniformity
Discussion: The guide describes the measurement of masking sound in an open office environment. The masking sound will usually be associated with a masking system, however, in certain positions and frequency ranges, HVAC equipment may affect or determine the masking sound spectrum. While intended primarily for open offices, this standard has been effectively used in closed, or mixed open and closed, offices.

ASTM E1110 - Classification for Determination of Articulation Class

Use: Provides a single figure rating that can be used for comparing building systems for speech privacy. The rating is designed to correlate with transmitted speech intelligence between office spaces.
Result: Articulation Class (AC)
Discussion: Weighting factors are applied to the one-third octave band attenuation data determined in Method E1111, E1375-90, and E1376-90. The weighted data are then totaled and rounded to the nearest multiple of 10 to yield the Articulation Class. A single number rating is convenient for ranking building materials and systems. However, for critical applications, a study of all available frequency data is advised to determine suitability.

ASTM E1111 - Test Method for Measuring the Interzone Attenuation of Ceiling Systems.

Use: Provides measurements of the sound reflective characteristics of ceiling systems when used in conjunction with partial-height space dividers.
Result: Interzone Attenuation and Articulation Class (AC)
Discussion: The ceiling system test specimen may include ceiling board, ceiling grid, lights, HVAC outlets, and related items. It is restricted to measurements with a fixed space divider height of 1.50 m (60 inches), a ceiling height of 2.7 m (108 inches), a sound source height of 1.20 m (48 inches), and microphone positions at 1.2 m of height. The interzone attenuation is the difference, in decibels, in a given one-third-octave band, between the measured reference level and the level measured at a nominal interzone distance. The preferred single number rating is the Articulation Class (AC) as described in ASTM E1110.

ASTM E1130-90 - Test Method for Objective Measurement of Speech Privacy in Open Offices Using Articulation Index.

Use: Field test of speech privacy in an open office. It can be used as a part of acceptance criteria for a completed office, or using a mock-up, may be helpful in predicting the privacy in a planned layout.
Result: Articulation Index (AI)
Discussion: The speech privacy between open offices is determined by the degree to which intruding speech sounds from adjacent offices exceed the ambient sound pressure levels at the listener's ear. This test method describes a means of measuring speech privacy objectively between locations in open offices. It relies upon acoustical measurements, published information on speech levels, and standard methods for assessing speech privacy. It measures the overall performance of the office; it is not a component test.

ASTM E1374-90 - Guide to Open Office Acoustics and Applicable ASTM Standards.

Use: This guide discusses the acoustical principles and interactions that affect the acoustical environment and acoustical privacy in the open office.
Result: Guidelines and suggestions
Discussion: This practice is intended for the use of architects, engineers, office managers and others interested in designing, specifying or operating open offices. A successful open plan office is the result of careful coordination of the several components - ceiling, wall treatments, furniture and furnishings, heating, ventilating and air-conditioning system and masking sound system. --the guide attempts to clarify the many interacting variables which influence office privacy, --.

ASTM E1375-90 - Test Method for Measuring the Interzone Attenuation of Furniture Panels used as Acoustical Barriers.

Use: Provides a measurement of the interzone attenuation (i.e. sound barrier characteristics) of furniture panels (screens or part high barriers) in open-plan spaces to provide speech privacy or sound isolation between working positions.
Result: Interzone attenuation and Articulation Class (AC)
Discussion: The part-high space divider specimen may be systems furniture panels, screens or the like installed in a typical in use configuration. The method measures the degree to which sound is diffracted over the top edge and transmitted through the panel. As with the companion ceiling test E1111, the procedure is restricted to measurements with a pre-determined ceiling at a fixed ceiling height of 2.7 m (108 inches), a sound source height of 1.2 m (48 inches), and microphone positions at 1.2 m of height. The barrier height and configuration may vary per design. The interzone attenuation is the difference, in decibels, in a given one-third-octave band, between the measured reference level and the level measured at a nominal interzone distance. The preferred single number rating is the Articulation Class (AC) as defined by ASTM E1111.

E1376-90 - Test Method for Measuring the Interzone Attenuation of Sound Reflected by Wall Finishes and Furniture Panels.

Use: -- measures the degree to which reflected sound is attenuated by the most commonly found vertical surfaces in open-plan spaces.
Result: Interzone Attenuation and Articulation Class (AC)
Discussion: The vertical surfaces covered by this standard include wall finishes, such as sound-absorbent panels, and furniture panels or screens. It does not cover such items as window finishes or furniture other than panels. A companion to ASTM E1375 and E1111 the test setup is identical with the exception that the specimen covers a portion of the test chamber wall in the flanking position such as may be found with a screen located perpendicular to a wall and spaced several feet away. The preferred single number rating is Articulation Class (AC).

(Proposed ASTM Standard) - Standard Method of Test for Airborne Sound Attenuation Between Rooms Sharing a Common Ceiling and Plenum.

Use: Measure the sound attenuation provided by a suspended ceiling in the presence of a continuous plenum space.

Result: Sound Transmission Class (STC)
Discussion: An adaptation of the well known AMA I-II, this method utilizes a laboratory space so arranged that it simulates a pair of horizontally adjacent small offices or rooms separated by a partition and sharing a common plenum space. -- the only significant sound transmission path is by way of the ceiling and the plenum space. This procedure is one of two methods to evaluate the acoustical performance of ceiling systems in an open/closed plan design, the other being E1111.

Table II

SUGGESTED ACOUSTICAL CRITERIA
FOR
AN OPEN/CLOSED OFFICE REQUIRING "CONFIDENTIAL SPEECH PRIVACY"

Environmental Element	Criteria	Test Reference
Ceiling system (including grid, lights, board and HVAC outlets)	AC > 220 STC > 40 Compliance	ASTM E1110 and E1111 ASTM proposed method ASTM C635 and E1264
Part high space divider (barrier position)	AC > 220	ASTM E1110 and E1375
Part high space divider (flanking position)	AC > 220	ASTM E1110 and E1376
Full high space divider (barrier position)	AC > 550	Revised version of ASTM E1110 and E1375
Full high space divider (flanking position)	AC > 220	ASTM E1110 and E1376
Wall and column covers	AC > 220	ASTM E1110 and E1376
Window walls	AC > 220	Revised version of ASTM E1110 and E1376
Raised floor systems	STC > 40	Inverted version of ceiling attenuation
Masking sound system	+/- 2 dB Spatial and Temporal Uniformity	ASTM E1041
Field evaluation of completed pair of typical work stations	AI > .05	ASTM E1130
Application of ceiling	Compliance	ASTM C635
Application of acoustical materials in general	Compliance	Expanded version of ASTM E1374

APPENDIX 1 - GLOSSARY OF ACOUSTICAL TERMS

(Note: These definitions are excerpted from ASTM C 634, Standard Definitions of Terms Relating to Environmental Acoustics. Those noted by an * are provided by NCA)

<u>Acoustical material</u> — any material considered in terms of its acoustical properties. **Commonly and especially, a material designed to absorb sound.**

<u>Airborne sound</u> — sound that arrives at the point of interest, such as one side of a partition, by propagation through air.

<u>Ambient noise</u> — the composite of airborne sound from many sources near and far associated with a given environment. No particular sound is singled out for interest.

<u>Average sound pressure level</u> — of several related sound pressure levels measured at different positions or different times, or both, in a specified frequency band, ten times the common logarithm of the arithmetic mean of the squared pressure ratios from which the individual levels were derived. Note: an average sound pressure level obtained by integrating and averaging during certain time periods is often called equivalent sound pressure level and, when A-weighted, equivalent sound level.

<u>Background noise</u> — noise from all sources unrelated to a particular sound that is the object of interest. Background noise may include airborne, structureborne, and instrument noise.

<u>Composite loss factor</u>* (CFL) — A measure of the damping characteristics of a material or system. Acceptable damping has a composite loss factor of 0.05.

<u>Damp</u> — to cause a loss or dissipation of the oscillatory or vibrational energy of an electrical or mechanical system.

<u>Decay rate</u> — for airborne sound, the rate of decrease of sound pressure level after the source of sound has stopped; for vibration, the rate of decrease of vibratory acceleration, velocity, or displacement level after the excitation has stopped.

<u>Decibel</u> (dB) — the term used to identify ten times the common logarithm of the ratio of two like quantities proportional to power or energy. (See level, sound transmission loss.) Thus, one decibel corresponds to a power ratio of (10 to the 0.1 power) to the n power. Note: since the decibel expresses the ratio of two like quantities, it has no dimensions. It is, however, common practice to treat "decibel" as a unit as, for example, in the sentence, "The average sound pressure level in the room is 45 decibels."

<u>Diffraction</u> — a change in the direction of propagation of sound energy in the neighborhood of a boundary discontinuity, such as the edge of a reflective or absorptive surface.

Diffuse sound field — the sound in a region where the intensity is the same in all directions and at every point.

Direct sound field — the sound that arrives directly from a source without reflection.

Field sound transmission class (FSTC) — a single-number rating derived from measured values of field transmission loss in accordance with Classification E 413, Determination of Sound Transmission Class. It provides an estimate of the performance of the partition in certain common sound insulation problems.

Field transmission loss (FTL) — of a partition installed in a building, in a specified frequency band, the ratio, expressed on the decibel scale, of the airborne sound power incident on the partition to the sound power transmitted by the partition and radiated on the other side.

Flanking transmission — transmission of sound from the source to a receiving location by a path other than that under consideration.

Frequency* — the number of cycles per second measured in units of Hertz (Hz). A frequency of 1000 Hz means 1000 cycles per second.

Impact insulation class (IIC) — a single-number rating derived from measured values of normalized impact sound pressure levels in accordance with Annex A1 of ASTM Method E 492, Laboratory Measurement of Impact Sound Transmission Through Floor-Ceiling Assemblies Using the Tapping Machine. It provides an estimate of the impact sound insulating performance of a floor-ceiling assembly.

Impact noise rating* (INR) — a single-number rating of a floor/ceiling assembly derived from measured values of impact noise when tested in accordance with procedure ISO R140 (Tapping Machine) This rating is similar to and replaced by IIC.

Insertion loss (IL) — of a silencer or other sound-reducing element, in a specified frequency band, the decrease in sound power level, measured at the location of the receiver, when a sound insulator or a sound attenuator is inserted in the transmission path between the source and the receiver.

Level (L) — ten times the common logarithm of the ratio of a quantity proportional to power or energy to a reference quantity of the same kind. (See sound power level, sound pressure level.) The quantity so obtained is expressed in decibels.

Level reduction (LR) — in a specified frequency band, the decrease in sound pressure level, measured at the location of the receiver, when a barrier or other sound-reducing element is placed between the source and the receiver. Note: level reduction is a useful measure in circumstances when transmission loss, insertion loss, or noise reduction are not measurable.

Metric sabin [L^2] — the unit of measure of sound absorption in the meter-kilogram-second system of units.

Noise isolation class (NIC) — a single-number rating derived from measured values of noise reduction, as though they were values of transmission loss, in accordance with ASTM Classification E 413, Determination of Sound Transmission Class. It provides an estimate of the sound isolation between two enclosed spaces that are acoustically connected.

Noise reduction (NR) — in a specified frequency band, the difference between the space-time average sound pressure levels produced in two enclosed spaces or rooms by one or more sound sources in one of them. Note: it is implied that in each room there is a meaningful average level; that is, that in each room the individual observations are randomly distributed about the average value, with no systematic variation with the position within the permissible measurement region. Noise reduction becomes meaningless and should not be used in situations where this condition is not met.

Noise reduction coefficient (NRC) — a single-number rating derived from measured values of sound absorption coefficients in accordance with ASTM Test Method C 423, for Sound Absorption and Sound Absorption Coefficients by the Reverberation Room Method. It provides an estimate of the sound absorptive property of an acoustical material. *NRC values range from near 0 for hard reflective materials such as glass and gypsum board to 1.2 for several inches of highly efficient fiberglass boards.

Normalized noise reduction (NNR) — between two rooms, for a specified frequency band, the value that the noise reduction in a given field test would have if the reverberation time in the receiving room were 0.5 seconds.

Normal mode — of a room, one of the possible ways in which the air in a room, considered as an elastic body, will vibrate naturally when subjected to an acoustical disturbance. With each normal mode is associated a resonance frequency and, in general, a group of wave propagation directions comprising a closed path.

Outdoor-indoor transmission loss (OITL) — of a building facade, in a specified frequency band, ten times the common logarithm of the ratio of the airborne sound power incident on the exterior of the facade to the sound power transmitted by the facade and radiated to the interior. The quantity so obtained is expressed in decibels.

Pink noise — noise with a continuous frequency spectrum and with equal power per constant percentage bandwidth. For example, equal power in any one-third octave band.

Receiving room — in architectural acoustical measurements, the room in which the sound transmitted from the source room is measured.

Reverberant sound field — the sound in an enclosed or partially enclosed space that has been reflected repeatedly or continuously from the boundaries.

Reverberation — the persistence of sound in an enclosed or partially enclosed space after the source of sound has stopped; by extension, in some contexts, the sound that so persists.

Reverberation room — a room so designed that the reverberant sound field closely approximates a diffuse sound field, both in the steady state when the sound source is on and during decay after the source of sound has stopped.

Sabin, $[L^2]$ — the unit of measure of sound absorption in the inch-pound system. (i.e. 1 sabin = 1 dB/square foot.)

Sound absorption — (1) the process of dissipating sound energy. (2) the property possessed by materials, objects and structures such as rooms of absorbing sound energy. (3) A; $[L_2]$; metric sabin - in a specified frequency band, the measure of the absorptive property of a material, an object, or a structure such as a room. Note: sound energy passing through a wall or opening may be regarded as being absorbed in certain calculations.

Sound absorption coefficient (α) (dimensionless); metric sabin/m^2 - of a surface, in a specified frequency band, the measure of the absorptive property of a material as approximated by the method of ASTM Test Method C 423, for Sound Absorption and Sound Absorption Coefficients by the Reverberation Room Method. Ideally, the fraction of the randomly incident sound power absorbed or otherwise not reflected.

Sound attenuation — the reduction of the intensity of sound as it travels from the source to a receiving location. Sound absorption is often involved as, for instance, in a lined duct. Spherical spreading and scattering or other attenuation mechanisms.

Sound insulation — the capacity of a structure to prevent sound from reaching a receiving location. Sound energy is not necessarily absorbed; impedance mismatch, or reflection back toward the source, is often the principal mechanism. Note: sound insulation is a matter of degree. No partition is a perfect insulator of sound.

Sound intensity (I): $[MT^3]$; W/m^2 — the quotient obtained when the average rate of energy flow in a specified direction and sense is divided by the area, perpendicular to that direction, through or toward which it flows. The intensity at a point is the limit of that quotient as the area that includes the point approaches zero.

Sound isolation — the degree of lack of acoustical connection. There are, in general, two ways to achieve a degree of sound isolation: by insulation, preventing the sound from reaching a receiving location, and by attenuation, reducing the intensity of sound as it travels toward a receiving location.

Sound level — of airborne sound, a sound pressure level obtained using a signal to which a standard frequency weighting has been applied. Note 1: three standard frequency-weightings designated A, B and C are defined in ANSI S1.4, Specification for Sound Level Meters. Note

2: the frequency-weighting and method of averaging must be specified unless clear from the context.

Sound power (W); $[ML^2T^3]$; (W) – in a specified frequency band, the rate at which acoustic energy is radiated from a source. In general, the rate of flow of sound energy, whether from a source, through and area, or into an absorber.

Sound power level (L_w) – of airborne sound, ten times the common logarithm of the ratio of the sound power under consideration to the standard reference power of 1 pW. The quantity so obtained is expressed in decibels.

Sound pressure (p); $[ML^{-1}T^{-2}]$; Pa – a fluctuating pressure superimposed on the static pressure by the presence of sound. In analogy with alternating voltage, its magnitude can be expressed in several ways, such as instantaneous sound pressure or peak sound pressure, but the unqualified term means root-mean-square sound pressure. In air, the static pressure is barometric pressure.

Sound pressure level (L_p) – of airborne sound, ten times the common logarithm of the ratio of the square of the sound pressure under consideration to the square of the standard reference pressure of 20 uPa. The quantity so obtained is expressed in decibels. Note: the pressures are squared because pressure squared, rather than pressure, is proportional to power or energy.

Sound transmission class (STC) – a single-number rating derived from measured values of transmission loss in accordance with ASTM Classification E 413, Determination of Sound Transmission Class. It provides an estimate of the performance of a partition in certain common sound insulation problems.

Sound transmission loss (TL) – of a partition, in a specified frequency band, ten times the common logarithm of the ratio of the airborne sound power incident on the partition to the sound power transmitted by the partition and radiated on the other side. The quantity so obtained is expressed in decibels. Note: unless qualified, the term denotes the sound transmission loss obtained when the specimen is exposed to a diffuse sound field as approximated, for example, in reverberation rooms meeting the requirements of ASTM Test Method E 90 for Laboratory Measurement of Airborne-sound Transmission Loss of Building Partitions.

Source room – in architectural acoustical measurements, the room that contains the noise source or sources.

Speech privacy noise isolation class* (NIC') – A single number rating system derived from data on a screen, ceiling, wall covering, background masking system or a complete interior environment (i.e. open plan office) using PBS C.2 test procedures. This is an objective measurement that is the forerunner of several ASTM standards for the open plan office.

Speech privacy potential* (SPP) — a single number rating system derived from the data generated by evaluating the sound attenuation characteristics of an office screen, ceiling, wall treatment, background masking system or a complete acoustical system using test method PBS C.1. This is a "subjective measurement" usually used in the field to evaluate the degree of speech privacy between two adjacent work stations.

Structureborne sound — sound that arrives at the point of interest, such as the edge of a partition, by propagation through a solid structure.

Vibration isolation — a reduction, attained by the use of a resilient coupling, in the capacity of a system to vibrate in response to mechanical excitation.

White noise — noise with a continuous frequency spectrum and with equal power per unit bandwidth. For example, equal power in any band of 100 Hz width.

****

APPENDIX 2 - ACOUSTICAL STANDARDS

The following organizations publish ACOUSTICAL consensus standards.

PREFIX	ORGANIZATION/address
AMA	Acoustical Materials Association (defunct) Contact: Ceiling & Interior Contractors Association 104 Wilmot Rd., Deerfield, IL 60015
ANSI	American National Standards Institute 1430 Broadway, New York, NY 10018
ARI	Air Conditioning and Refrigeration Institute 1815 N. Ft. Myer Dr., Arlington, VA 22209
ASA	Acoustical Society of America (Standards Secretariat/Journal - ASA & ISO) 335 East 45th Street, New York, NY 10017
ASHRAE	American Society of Heating, Refrigerating and Air-Conditioning Engineers 1791 Tullie Circle, N.E., Atlanta, GA 30329
ASTM	American Society of Testing & Materials (Book of Standards Volume 04.06) 1916 Race St., Philadelphia, PA 19103 (Environmental Acoustics)
IEEE	Institute of Electrical and Electronic Engineers 345 East 47th Street, New York, NY 10017
ISA	Instrument Society of America P.O. Box 12277, 67 Alexander Dr., Research Triangle Park, NC 27709
ISO/IEC	International Organization for Standardization International Electrotechnical Commission 1 Rue de Varembe, Case Postale 56, CH-1211 Geneva 20, Switzerland
NCA	Noise Control Association 104 Cresta Verde Dr., Rolling Hills Est., CA 90274
NEMA	National Electrical Manufacturers Association 2101 L Street N.W., Washington, DC 20037

NFPA	National Fluid Power Association P.O. Box 49, Thiensville, WI 53092
NMTBA	National Machine Tool Builders Association 7901 West Park Drive, McLean, VA 22102
SAE	Society of Automotive Engineers 400 Commonwealth Drive, Warrendale, PA 15096

STANDARDS AND PROCEDURES (Related to Acoustics)

The following is a listing and a brief synopsis, where available, of the standard. Please reference the standard for additional details. The descriptions for ASTM Standards were excerpted from ASTM E1374-90, "Guide to Standards of ASTM Technical Committee E-33 on Environmental Acoustics." Other descriptions were prepared by NCA. For additional information or clarification, ASTM E-33 Sub-Committee jurisdiction is as follows:

- E33.01 - Sound Absorption
- E33.02 - Open Plan Spaces
- E33.03 - Sound Transmission
- E33.04 - Application
- E33.05 - Research
- E33.06 - International Standards
- E33.07 - Definitions and Editorial
- E33.08 - Mechanical and Electrical System Noise
- E33.09 - Community Noise

(NOTE: This listing is for information purposes only. Please reference each individual standard for proper use, limits and related concerns. NCA assumes no risk or responsibility for improper utilization of these standards.)

SOUND POWER AND LEVEL MEASUREMENT

ANSI S1.13 — Standard Methods for the Measurement of Sound Pressure Levels (1976)

ISO 3740 — Determination of Sound Power Levels of Noise Sources - Guidelines for Use of Basic Standards and Preparation of Noise Test Codes (1978)

ISO 3741 — Determination of Sound Power Levels of Noise Sources - Precision Methods for Broad-Band Sound Sources Operating in Reverberation Rooms (1975)

ISO 3742 — Determination of Sound Power Levels of Noise Sources - Precision Methods for Discrete-Frequency and Narrow-Band Sound Sources Operating in Reverberation Rooms (1975)

ISO 3744 — Determination of Sound Power Levels of Noise Sources - Engineering Methods for Free-Field Conditions over a Reflecting Plane

ISO 3745 — Determination of Sound Power Levels of Noise Sources - Precision Methods for Sources Operating in Anechoic Rooms

ISO 3746 — Determination of Sound Power Levels of Noise Sources - Survey Method

ISO 3747 — Determination of Sound Power Levels of Noise Sources - Methods Using a Reference Sound Source

ANSI S3.17 — Method for Rating the Sound Power Spectra of Small Stationary Noise Sources

ANSI S1.21 — Standard Methods for the Determination of Sound Power Levels of Small Sources in Reverberation Rooms (1976)

ANSI S3.4 — Standard Procedure for the Computation of Loudness of Noise (1972)

ANSI S3.5 — Methods for the Calculation of the Articulation Index (1976)

ACOUSTICAL MEASUREMENT/METER STANDARDS

IEC (ISO) 179 — Precision Sound Level Meters (1973)

IEC (ISO) 179A — Additional Characteristics for the Measurement of Impulsive Sounds (1973)

IEC (ISO) 225 — Octave, Half-Octave and Third-Octave Band Filters Intended for the Analysis of Sounds and Vibrations (1966)

IEC (ISO) 327 — Precision Method for the Pressure Calibration of One-Inch Standard Condenser Microphones by the Reciprocity Technique (1971)

IEC (ISO) 402 — Simplified Methods for Pressure Calibration of One Inch Condenser Microphones by the Reciprocity Technique (1972)

ANSI S1.2 — Method for the Physical Measurement of Sound (1976)

ANSI S1.4 — Specification for Sound Level Meters (1971)

ANSI S1.6 – Preferred Frequencies and Band Numbers for Acoustical Measurements (1976)

ANSI S1.8 – Preferred Reference Quantities for Acoustical Levels (1974)

ANSI S1.10 – Method for the Calibration of Microphones (1976)

ANSI S1.11 – Specification for Octave, Half-Octave, and Third-Octave Band Filter Sets (1976)

ANSI S1.12 – Specifications for Laboratory Standard Microphones (1972)

SOUND ABSORPTION STANDARDS

ASTM C384 – Test Method for Impedance and Absorption of Acoustical Materials by the Impedance Tube Method

Use: Intended primarily as a research screening tool, useful for manufacturers and/or researchers in evaluating the absorption of materials. It is also valuable for evaluating small units, such as anechoic wedges. It can be used to rank order the absorption and impedance characteristics of materials.
Result: Normal Incidence Sound Absorption Coefficients, Normal Specific Impedance Ratios
Discussion: A sound wave traveling down a tube is reflected back by the test specimen, producing a standing wave that can be explored with a probe microphone. The normal absorption coefficient is determined from the standing wave ratio. In addition, an impedance ratio at any one frequency can be determined using the position of the standing wave with reference to the face of the specimen (See also Test Method E1050). Values do not necessarily correlate with those of C423.

ASTM C423 – Test Method for Sound Absorption and Sound Absorption Coefficients by the Reverberation Room Method

Use: Primary method for evaluating sound absorption capabilities of building materials and systems. One can use the sound absorption coefficients and volume of a room, or Sabins per unit, to determine how much material is needed to limit room reverberation and/or reduce noise to a desired level.
Result: Sound Absorption Coefficients, Noise Reduction Coefficient (NRC), Absorption figures in Sabins, Sabins/Unit
Discussion: Random noise is turned on long enough for the sound pressure in a reverberant room to reach a steady state. When the signal is turned off, the sound pressure level decreases. The rate of decrease (decay) in a specified frequency band is measured. The absorption of the room and its contents is calculated both before and after placing the specimen in the room. The increase in absorption due to the specimen, divided by the area of the specimen is the absorption coefficient. Noise Reduction Coefficient is the average of the four absorption coefficients of the third-octave bands centered on 250, 500, 1000 and 2000

Hz, rounded to the nearest .05. NRC is a single number rating and is convenient for ranking building materials and systems. However, in some critical applications, study of all available frequency data is advised to determine suitability.

ASTM C522 – Test Method for Airflow Resistance of Acoustical Material

Use: Indicates sound absorbing properties in some materials where airflow resistance is related to sound absorption.
Result: Airflow resistance (R), Specific Airflow resistance (r), Airflow resistivity (r_0)
Discussion: The specific airflow resistance of an acoustical material is one of the properties that determine its sound-absorptive and sound-transmitting properties. The specific air flow resistance is given by the formula R = P/U, where P = air pressure difference across the specimen, U = volume velocity of airflow through it. The specific airflow resistance measured by this method may differ from the specific resistance measured by the impedance tube method in Test Method C384. *Caution : materials exist that do not allow any airflow yet exhibit excellent sound absorption.*

ASTM E795 – Practices for Mounting Test Specimens During Sound Absorption Tests

Use: Reference to specific mounting methods helps laboratory operators simulate expected field applications. It also helps specifiers by allowing comparison of materials tested in similar mountings.
Result: A letter designation describing the method of mounting a C423 test specimen.
Discussion: These practices cover test specimen mountings to be used during tests performed in accordance with Test Method C423. Sound absorption of a material covering a flat surface depends not only on the physical properties of the material, but also on the way in which the material is mounted over the surface. The mountings specified in these practices are intended to simulate, in the laboratory, conditions that exist in normal use.

ASTM E1042 – Classification for Acoustically Absorptive Materials Applied by Trowel or Spray

Use: This standard helps specifiers select materials by classifying certain characteristics.
Result: Classification of materials
Discussion: Acoustically absorptive materials are used for the control of reverberation and echoes in rooms. This standard provides a classification method for such materials applied directly to surfaces by trowel or by spray. Classification is made according to type of material: acoustical absorption determined by C423, flame spread determined by E84, and dust propensity determined by E859.

ASTM E1050 – Test Method for Impedance and Absorption of Acoustical Materials Using a Tube, Two Microphones, and a Digital Frequency Analysis System

Use: Intended primarily as a research tool. This is an alternative to C384 using digital instruments.
Result: Normal Incidence Sound Absorption Coefficients, Normal Specific Acoustic Impedance Ratios
Discussion: A broadband noise is produced on one end of a tube, the other end of which contains a test specimen. The plane wave produced is detected by two microphones located at different positions along the tube. A digital frequency analyzer measures the output from the two microphones. Results match closely with C384.

OPEN OFFICE ACOUSTICAL STANDARDS

ASTM E1041 – Guide for Measurement of Masking Sound in Open Offices

Use: Measures variation of masking sound over time and throughout a space, and its correlation to a specified sound spectrum. Can be used as an acceptance or problem solving tool by specifiers.
Result: Spatial and Temporal Uniformity
Discussion: The guide describes the measurement of masking sound in an open office environment. The masking sound will usually be associated with a masking system, however, in certain positions and frequency ranges, HVAC equipment may affect or determine the masking sound spectrum. While intended primarily for open offices, this standard has been effectively used in closed, or mixed open and closed, offices.

ASTM E1110 – Classification for Determination of Articulation Class

Use: Provides a single figure rating that can be used for comparing building systems for speech privacy. The rating is designed to correlate with transmitted speech intelligence between office spaces.
Result: Articulation Class (AC)
Discussion: Weighting factors are applied to the one-third octave band attenuation data determined in Method E1111, E1375-90, and E1376-90. The weighted data are then totaled and rounded to the nearest multiple of 10 to yield the Articulation Class. A single number rating is convenient for ranking building materials and systems. However, for critical applications, a study of all available frequency data is advised to determine suitability.

ASTM E1111 – Test Method for Measuring the Interzone Attenuation of Ceiling Systems

Use: Provides measurements of the sound reflective characteristics of ceiling systems when used in conjunction with partial-height space dividers.
Result: Interzone Attenuation and Articulation Class (AC)
Discussion: The ceiling system test specimen may include ceiling board, ceiling grid, lights, HVAC outlets, and related items. It is restricted to measurements with a fixed space divider height of 1.50 m (60 inches), a ceiling height of 2.7 m (108 inches), a sound source height of 1.20 m (48 inches) and microphone positions at 1.2 m of height. The interzone attenuation

is the difference, in decibels, in a given one-third-octave band, between the measured reference level and the level measured at a nominal interzone distance. The preferred single number rating is the Articulation Class (AC) as described in ASTM E1110.

ASTM E1130-90 – Test Method for Objective Measurement of Speech Privacy in Open Offices Using Articulation Index

Use: Field test of speech privacy in an open office. It can be used as a part of acceptance criteria for a completed office, or using a mock-up, may be helpful in predicting the privacy in a planned layout.
Result: Articulation Index (AI)
Discussion: The speech privacy between open offices is determined by the degree to which intruding speech sounds from adjacent offices exceed the ambient sound pressure levels at the listener's ear. This test method describes a means of measuring speech privacy objectively between locations in open offices. It relies upon acoustical measurements, published information on speech levels, and standard methods for assessing speech privacy. It measures the overall performance of the office; it is not a component test.

ASTM E1374-90 – Guide to Open Office Acoustics and Applicable ASTM Standards

Use: This guide discusses the acoustical principles and interactions that affect the acoustical environment and acoustical privacy in the open office.
Result: Guidelines and suggestions
Discussion: This practice is intended for the use of architects, engineers, office managers and others interested in designing, specifying or operating open offices. A successful open plan office is the result of careful coordination of the several components – ceiling, wall treatments, furniture and furnishings, heating, ventilating and air-conditioning system and masking sound system. The guide attempts to clarify the many interacting variables which influence office privacy.

ASTM E1375-90 – Test Method for Measuring the Interzone Attenuation of Furniture Panels Used as Acoustical Barriers

Use: Provides a measurement of the interzone attenuation (i.e. sound barrier characteristics) of furniture panels (screens or part high barriers) in open-plan spaces to provide speech privacy or sound isolation between working positions.
Result: Interzone attenuation and Articulation Class (AC)
Discussion: The part high space divider specimen may be systems furniture panels, screens or the like installed in a typical in use configuration. The method measures the degree to which sound is diffracted over the top edge and transmitted through the panel. As with the companion ceiling test E1111, the procedure is restricted to measurements with a predetermined ceiling at a fixed ceiling height of 2.7 m (108 inches), a sound source height of 1.2 m (48 inches), and microphone positions at 1.2 m of height. The barrier height and configuration may vary per design. The interzone attenuation is the difference, in decibels,

in a given one-third-octave band, between the measured reference level and the level measured at a nominal interzone distance. The preferred single number rating is the Articulation Class (AC) as defined by ASTM E1111.

ASTM E1376-90 — Test Method for Measuring the Interzone Attenuation of Sound Reflected by Wall Finishes and Furniture Panels

Use: Measures the degree to which reflected sound is attenuated by the most commonly found vertical surfaces in open-plan spaces.
Result: Interzone Attenuation and Articulation Class (AC)
Discussion: The vertical surfaces covered by this standard include wall finishes, such as sound-absorbent panels, and furniture panels or screens. It does not cover such items as window finishes or furniture other than panels. A companion to ASTM E1375 and E1111 the test setup is identical with the exception that the specimen covers a portion of the test chamber wall in the flanking position such as may be found with a screen located perpendicular to a wall and spaced several feet away. The preferred single number rating is Articulation Class (AC).

SOUND TRANSMISSION STANDARDS

AMA I-II and ASTM E-1414 ▪ Standard — Standard Method of Test for Airborne Sound Attenuation Between Rooms Sharing a Common Ceiling and Plenum

Use: Measure the sound attenuation provided by a suspended ceiling in the presence of a continuous plenum space.
Result: Sound Transmission Class (STC)
Discussion: The ASTM version is an adaptation of the well known AMA I-II. This method utilizes a laboratory space so arranged that it simulates a pair of horizontally adjacent small offices or rooms separated by a partition and sharing a common plenum space. The only significant sound transmission path is by way of the ceiling and the plenum space. This procedure is one of two methods to evaluate the acoustical performance of ceiling systems in an open/closed plan design, the other being E1111.

ASTM E90 — Test Method for Laboratory Measurement of Airborne Sound Transmission Loss of Building Partitions

Use: Primary method for evaluating transmission loss of materials and systems used in building construction, such as interior partitions, doors, windows, and floor/ceiling assemblies.
Result: Transmission Loss (TL)
Discussion: A test specimen is installed in an opening between two adjacent reverberation rooms, care being taken that the only significant sound path between rooms is by way of the specimen. An approximately diffuse field is produced in one room, and the resulting space-

time average sound pressure levels in the two rooms are determined at a number of one-third-octave band frequencies. In addition, the sound absorption in the receiving room is determined. The sound transmission loss is calculated from a basic relationship involving difference between the sound levels, the receiving room absorption, and the test specimen size. The TL data are used in E413 to Determine Sound Transmission Class (STC).

ASTM E336 – Test Method for Measurement of Airborne Sound Insulation in Buildings

Use: Primary method for evaluating on-site noise reduction between two rooms or sound barrier performance of interior partitions. Can be used for acceptance of recent construction or improvement of existing buildings. It is not recommended to use test performance in one facility to predict results in another.
Result: Field Transmission Loss (FTL), Noise Reduction (NR), Normalized Noise Reduction (NNR)
Discussion: The noise reduction between two rooms is obtained by taking the difference between the average sound pressure levels in each room at specified frequencies in one-third-octave bands when one room contains a noise source. The noise reduction may be normalized to a reference reverberation time of 0.5 seconds. When the rooms' size and absorption requirements are satisfied so that the sound fields are sufficiently diffuse and when flanking is not significant, the field transmission loss may be reported. Results will usually be lower than in E90 laboratory tests for the same specimen. Note that this test requires minimum room characteristics to be valid (see also Method E597). The data are used in E413 to Determine Noise Isolation Class (NIC), Normalized Noise Isolation Class (NNIC), or Field Sound Transmission Class (FSTC).

ASTM E413 – Classification for Rating Sound Insulation

Use: Permits specifiers to rank the transmission loss or noise reduction performance of similar materials or systems, using data from one of several test methods.
Result: Sound Transmission Class (STC), Field Sound Transmission Class (FSTC), Noise Isolation Class (NIC), Normalized Noise Isolation Class (NNIC)
Discussion: To determine the Sound Transmission Class (STC) of a test specimen, its transmission loss (as determined in accordance with Method E90), Field Transmission Loss (E336), Noise Reduction (E336 or E596), or Normalized Noise Reduction (E336) in a series of 16 test bands, are compared with those of a reference contour. When certain conditions are met, the Class is found. It is recommended that the test data be presented in a graph together with the corresponding Class contour. The single number rating is convenient for ranking building materials and systems. However, it is appropriate only for commonly found indoor sounds similar to speech. For critical applications, study of all available frequency data is advised to determine suitability.

ASTM E597 – Practice for Determining a Single-Number Rating of Airborne Sound Isolation for Use in Multiunit Building Specifications

Use: Determines the degree of acoustical isolation between and within dwelling units in apartment buildings, hotels, etc.
Result: Sound Level Difference (D), Normalized Sound Level Difference (D_n), Average Sound Level (L)
Discussion: The sound level difference between two rooms is measured by establishing a sound field with specified spectrum in a source room, of sufficient level that the corresponding sound in a receiving room predominates over the sound from all other sources. With the sound source in operation, the space-time average A-weighted sound level, L, in each of the two rooms, is measured. The difference between the levels is the sound level difference, D, for that room pair. (This value may vary from the Noise Isolation Class (NIC); see E336.) The sound level difference is a property of the two rooms and their contents, not of the dividing partition alone. Results will be lower than those found in E90, since flanking paths and imperfections are not eliminated from the test.

ASTM E756 – Method for Measuring Vibration-Damping Properties of Materials

Use: This method determines the vibration-damping properties of materials.
Results: Young's Modulus (E), Loss Factor (LF), Shear Modulus (G)
Discussion: This method is accurate over a frequency range of 50 to 5000 Hz and over the useful temperature range of the material being tested. It is useful in testing materials that have application in structural vibration, building acoustics, and the control of audible noise. Such materials include metals, enamels, ceramics, rubbers, plastics, reinforced epoxy matrices, and woods that can be formed to the test specimen configurations.

ASTM E966 – Guide for Field Measurement of Airborne Sound Insulation of Building Facades and Facade Elements

Use: Field test guide for measuring noise isolation of exterior walls and facade components.
Result: Outdoor-Indoor Transmission Loss (OITL), Outdoor-Indoor Level Reduction (OILR)
Discussion: Loudspeaker or traffic sound sources may be used. The outdoor sound field may be inferred from pre-calibration, or measured on site near the facade or at the facade surface. A fixed sound source is located at a specific angle, while traffic may move along a straight line in front of the facade. Indoors, a space average is taken in the room adjacent to the test facade. The difference between the two sound levels is OILR. (For uncontrolled sound sources and traffic, the outdoor and indoor sound levels are measured simultaneously.) To obtain OITL, OILR is normalized for room absorption, and flanking transmission paths must be blocked. If flanking transmission is present or unknown, the measurement is labeled the "apparent OITL" and represents the lower limit of noise isolation performance. Because of angle of incidence and flanking effects, results may not agree with those obtained with other test methods, such as E90 or E336.

ASTM E1123 – Practices for Mounting Test Specimens for Sound Transmission Loss Testing of Naval and Marine Ship Bulkhead Treatment Materials

Use: Provides laboratory operators with methods to mount test specimens to best reflect their application in actual shipboard use.
Purpose: To standardize mounting methods
Discussion: These practices describe test specimen mountings to be used for naval and marine ship applications during sound transmission loss tests performed in accordance with Method E90. The sound transmission loss of a material covering a flat surface depends partially upon the structure to which it is mounted and the mounting method used. Naval architects require specific transmission loss characteristics of acoustical treatment materials as they will be used on board ships.

ASTM E1332 – Classification for Determination of Outdoor-Indoor Transmission Class

Use: Provides a single-number rating to be used to compare building facade designs, including walls, doors, windows, and combinations thereof. The rating can be used by specifiers to rank-order building materials.
Result: Outdoor-Indoor Transmission Class (OITC)
Discussion: Using Transmission Loss Data in the range of 80 Hz to 4000 Hz, as measured in accordance with Method E90 or Guide E966, the OITC is calculated by applying A-weighting criteria to the reference source sound spectrum or source room sound levels, and subtracting the transmission loss. The resulting data are used in a provided formula to yield OITC. A sample manual worksheet and a computer program in the BASIC language are provided to help in applying the classification.

ASTM E596 – Test Method for Laboratory Measurement of the Noise Reduction of Sound-Isolating Enclosures

Use: Evaluating personnel enclosures to be used in noisy environments.
Result: Noise Reduction (NR)
Discussion: The enclosure to be tested is placed in a reverberation room and prepared for testing. The background noise levels inside the enclosure and in the reverberation room are measured in one-third octave-bands. After bands of random noise are produced in the reverberation room, the sound pressure levels are measured at several points in the reverberation room and at appropriate points inside the enclosure. The noise reduction in each one-third-octave band is the difference between the space-time-averaged sound pressure level in the reverberation room and the space-time-averaged sound pressure level inside the enclosure. The Noise Isolation Class (NIC) may be determined from the data using E413.

ASTM E1408 ▪ Standard Practice for Testing Transmission Loss of Doors and Door Seals

Use: Procedure for installing doors and seals in E90
Result: Procedure only - establishes the requirements for installation

IMPACT NOISE OF FLOORS

ASTM E492 – Method of Laboratory Measurement of Impact Sound Transmission Through Floor-Ceiling Assemblies Using the Tapping Machine

Use: This is the primary laboratory method for evaluating floor/ceiling assemblies as barriers to structure-borne rather than airborne noise. The standard tapping machine does not duplicate human footfall noise.
Result: Normalized Impact Sound Pressure Levels (L_n)
Discussion: A standard tapping machine is placed in operation on a test-floor specimen that forms a horizontal separation between two rooms, one directly above the other. The transmitted impact sound characterized by the spectrum of the space-time-average one-third-octave band sound pressure levels produced by the tapping machine is measured in the receiving room below. Since the spectrum depends on the absorption of the receiving room, the sound pressure levels are normalized to a reference absorption. Resulting data are used in E989 to determine Impact Isolation Class (ICC).

ASTM E989 – Classification for Determination of Impact Insulation Class (IIC)

Use: Provides single-number rating of the barrier capabilities of floor-ceiling assemblies against structure-borne noise.
Result: Impact Insulation Class (IIC), Field Impact Insulation Class (FLIC)
Discussion: The one-third octave laboratory impact noise data obtained in Method E492 or field data obtained in Method E1007, are compared with those of a reference contour. When certain conditions are met, the Class is found. It is recommended that the test data be presented in a graph together with the corresponding Class Contour. A single number rating is convenient for ranking building materials and systems. However, for critical applications, study of all available frequency data is advised to determine suitability.

ASTM E1007 – Test Method for Field Measurement of Tapping Machine Impact Sound Transmission Through Floor-Ceiling Assemblies and Associated Support Structures

Use: Measures transmission of impact sound generated by a standard tapping machine through floor/ceiling assemblies and associated supporting structures in field situations. Can be an acceptance or improvement tool for specifiers.
Result: Normalized Impact Sound Pressure Levels (L_n)
Discussion: Measurements may be conducted on all types of floor/ceiling assemblies, including those with floating-floor or suspended ceiling elements, or both, and assemblies surfaced with any type of floor surfaces or coverings. This field method does not distinguish between sound transmitted through the entire building and that transmitted solely through the floor/ceiling assemblies. The standard tapping machine does not duplicate human footfall noise. Because room sizes and shapes can vary widely, it is preferable to confine the use of

test results to the comparison of closely similar floors and supporting structures. Resulting data are used in E989 to determine Impact Isolation Class (IIC).

AMA I-I — Impact Sound Transmission Test by the Footfall Method

Use: This procedure was developed specifically to evaluate actual footfall sounds being transmitted to the receiver room below.
Result: Footstep sounds transmitted to rooms located directly below are masked by an acoustical environment of not greater than $NC_{40} = 40$ or 35.
Discussion: Either a male or female walker may be utilized with their size weight and footware carefully identified. It is applicable to both the laboratory and field. Since AMA no longer exists, copies of the procedure may be obtained from Geiger and Hamme Laboratories, Ann Arbor, MI, or the Ceiling and Insulating Systems Contractors Association (CISCA). This procedure evaluates the full spectrum of frequencies prevalent in a person walking. It does not correlate with the tapping machine tests leaving one to speculate which is appropriate. AMA I-I was designed and successfully measures actual field conditions.

APPLICATION STANDARDS

ASTM C367 — Test Methods for Strength Properties of Prefabricated Architectural Acoustical Tile or Lay-in Ceiling Panels

Use: This standard, when used in conjunction with tests of acoustic performance, helps specifiers select materials with the best combination of acoustic and strength properties for an intended application.
Result: Hardness, Friability, Sag, Transverse Strength
Discussion: Materials used for absorbing sound often have a porous, low-density structure and may be relatively fragile. These test methods cover procedures for evaluating those physical properties related to strength. The methods are useful in developing, manufacturing, and selecting acoustical tile or lay-in panels.

ASTM C635 — Specification for Metal Suspension Systems for Acoustical Tile and Lay-in Panel Ceilings

Use: This specification allows specifiers to evaluate and compare the physical characteristics of metal suspension systems.
Purpose: To aid in selecting materials
Discussion: This specification sets forth suspension member tolerances, load tests, and finish tests, to guide manufacturers and specifiers on acceptable products, and to give users and designers comparative test data to choose appropriate products.

ASTM C636 – Practice for Installation of Metal Ceiling Suspension Systems for Acoustical Tile and Lay-in Panels

Use: This practice is intended to be referenced by architects, designers, and/or owners of buildings.
Purpose: to aid in selecting materials
Discussion: This practice presents guidelines to designers and installers of acoustical ceilings and to other trades if their work interferes with ceiling components. Practices concerning hangers, carrying channels, main runners, cross runners, spline, assembly devices, and ceiling fixtures are discussed. Where seismic restraint is required, E580 should also be consulted, along with industry recommendations.

ASTM E497 – Practice for Installing Sound-isolating Lightweight Partitions

Use: Architects, designers, builders, and owners utilize this practice to assure fixed partition systems are free of major noise flanking paths and unnecessary leaks.
Purpose: to aid in design and specification
Discussion: This practice details precautions that should be taken during the installation of gypsum board partitions to maximize their sound insulating effectiveness. Potential problems with flanking sound transmission and sound leaks are discussed, and methods to avoid these are offered. A number of figures and drawings are included to illustrate the potential errors and to provide suggested precautions.

ASTM E557 – Practice for Architectural Application and Installation of Operable Partitions

Use: Architects, designers, builders, and owners utilize this practice to assure operable partition systems are free of major noise flanking paths and unnecessary leaks.
Purpose: to aid in design and specification
Discussion: This practice details precautions that must be taken before and during the installation of an operable partition to ensure that the maximum attainable sound insulation is achieved between the two spaces separated by the partition. Specific paragraphs refer to potential sound leakage through the partition joints, the seals, the ceiling and plenum, an HVAC system, and through hollow floors. Other paragraphs deal with deflection of the partition and potential problem of sound focusing by curved surfaces.

ASTM E580 – Practice for Application of Ceiling Suspension System for Acoustical Tile and Lay-in Panels in Areas Requiring Seismic Restraint

Use: This practice is an extension of Practice C636 and is intended to be referenced by architects, designers, and/or owners of buildings. It is critical in areas affected by earthquakes or tremors. Refer to local codes.
Purpose: to aid in design and specification
Discussion: This practice presents guidelines for designers and installers to provide additional restraint required in areas deemed by local authorities to be subject to major

seismic disturbance. Acceptable suspension system components, additional attachment points, and support elements for seismic restraint are described. Sketches show additional hanger wire locations and attachment. Specification C635 and Practice C636 cover suspension systems and their application, without regard to seismic restraint needs. *Building codes and manufacturers recommendations remain applicable and should be followed when this practice is specified.*

ASTM E1264 — Classification for Acoustical Ceiling Products

Use: This classification is intended to serve a similar purpose to Federal Specification SS-S-118B. Fire endurance and physical properties are not covered.
Result: Classification by acoustical, light reflectance, and surface burning characteristics.
Discussion: This classification covers ceiling products that provide acoustical performance and interior finish to buildings. It serves to classify and aid in the selection of acoustical ceiling products. Products are categorized by type, pattern, light reflectance, acoustical properties, and surface burning characteristics.

MECHANICAL AND ELECTRICAL SYSTEM NOISE STANDARDS

ASTM E477 — Test Method of Measuring Acoustical and Airflow Performance of Duct Liner Materials and Prefabricated Silencers

Use: This method applies to heating and air-conditioning ducts in buildings with low pressure and air speed.
Result: Insertion Loss (IL), Airflow-generated Sound Power Levels
Discussion: The sound pressure level in a reverberation room is measured while sound is entering the room through a length of straight, empty duct and again, after a section of the empty duct has been replaced with the test specimen. The insertion loss is the difference between the two sound pressure levels. Airflow-generated noise is measured while air is passing through the system with the specimen installed. Pressure drop performance is obtained by measuring the static pressure at designated locations upstream and downstream of the test specimen at various air flow settings.

ASTM E1124 — Test Method for Field Measurement of Sound Power Level by the Two-Surface Method

Use: Provides an estimate of the normal sound power level of a specimen operating in situ.
Result: Sound power level (L_w)
Discussion: The average one-third or full octave band sound pressure levels are measured over two different surfaces which surround the specimen. These surfaces should be selected to consist of rectangular, cylindrical, and/or hemispherical surfaces so that the areas may be easily calculated. From the difference between the two average sound pressure levels and from the areas of the surfaces the sound power level may be calculated. The calculation accounts for both the effect of the reverberant field and the noise of other sources.

ASTM E1265 — Test Method for Measuring Insertion Loss of Pneumatic Exhaust Silencers

Use: This standard permits specifiers to evaluate and compare the performance of pneumatic exhaust silencers.
Result: Flow Ratio, Average Insertion Loss
Discussion: This method covers the laboratory measurement of both the acoustical and mechanical performance of pneumatic exhaust silencers designed for quieting compressed gas exhausts from orifices up to 3/4" NPT. The method is not applicable for exhausts performing useful work, such as part conveying, ejection, or cleaning. The method evaluates acoustical performance using A-weighted sound level measurements.

ANSI S5.1 — Standard Test Code for the Measurement of Sound from Pneumatic Equipment (1971)

ASA 3-1975 — Test-Site Measurement of Noise Emitted by Engine Powered Equipment

ASHRAE 36-72 — Methods of Testing for Sound Rating Heating, Refrigerating, and Air-Conditioning Equipment (supersedes ASHRAE 36-72, 36A-63 and 36B-63)

IEEE 85 — Test Procedure for Airborne Sound Measurements on Rotating Electric Machinery (1973)

SAE J336a — Sound Level for Truck Cab Interior (1973)

SAE J672a — Exterior Loudness Evaluation of Heavy Trucks and Buses (1970)

SAE J952b — Sound Levels for Engine Powered Equipment (1969)

SAE J986a — Sound Level for Passenger Cars and Light Trucks (1973) (ANSI S6.3)

SAE J88a — Exterior Sound Level Measurement Procedure for Power Mobile Construction Machinery (1973)

AMCA 300-67 — Test Code for Sound Rating

AGMA 293.03 — Specification for Measurement of Sound on High Speed Helical and Herringbone Bear Units (1968)

AFBMA 13 — Rolling Bearing Vibration and Noise (1968)

AHAM RAC-2SR — Room Air Conditioner Sound Rating (1971)

DEMA — Test Case for the Measurement of Sound from Heavy-Duty Reciprocating Engine

NEMA MG1-12.49 — Motors and Generators - Methods of Measuring Machine Noise (1972)

NEMA TR1-1972 — Transformers, Regulators and Reactors - Section 9-04, Audible Sound Level Tests.

NFPA TS.9.70.12 — Method of Measuring Sound Generated by Hydraulic Fluid Power Pumps (1970)

NFPA T3.9.14 — Method of Measuring Sound Generated by Hydraulic Fluid Power Motors (1971)

NMBTA Technique — Noise Measurement Techniques (1970)

COMMUNITY NOISE STANDARDS

ASTM E1014 — Guide for Measurement of Outdoor A-Weighted Sound Levels

Use: Results from this guide may appropriately be used in conjunction with ordinances or land-use restrictions of noise by communities.
Result: A-weighted sound levels
Discussion: This guide covers measurement of A-weighted sound levels outdoors at specified locations or along particular site boundaries, using a general purpose sound-level meter. Three distinct types of measurement surveys are described: around a site boundary; at a specified location; and at a specified distance from a source (to find the maximum sound level). Since outdoor sound levels usually vary with time over a wide range, the data obtained using this guide may be presented in the form of a histogram of sound levels. The data obtained using this guide enables calculations of average or statistical sound levels for comparison with appropriate criteria.

DEFINITIONS OF ENVIRONMENTAL ACOUSTIC TERMS

ASTM C634 — Terminology Relating to Environmental Acoustics

Use: All other standards rely on these definitions. The user may need these definitions to understand a specific standard.
Result: Understanding of acoustic terms
Discussion: Definitions of terms used in Environmental Acoustics standards are provided, including, in those entries with physical properties, the symbol, dimensions, and units. (Many of the terms are contained in Appendix 1 of this manual.)

SUMMARY

This appendix provides a detail listing of all the acoustical standards published by industry organizations and consensus standards writing groups. This list contains all those standards known to the author and are well known in the United States of America. However, there are likely many others that are applicable.

****

Appendix 3 - DESIGN GUIDE and WORKSHEETS

Calculating acoustical predictors is both an art and a science. It has been the desire of every acoustician and person confronted with a noise problem to come up with a magical formula that will provide a good indicator of the resultant noise level after treatment. Unfortunately, there is no universal formula, though many have been postulated. A main concern of practical acousticians is that there are so many conditions that can change the results dramatically that it is nearly impossible to cover all circumstances. The following examples are given as an aid to selecting a design that may be practical for a particular set of circumstances. It is strongly urged that laboratory testing and field analysis be conducted if a specific criteria is to be satisfied. *While the following examples have been utilized successfully, NCA cannot assure their accuracy. If compliance with a specification, code or government criteria is required, it is recommended that a member of the National Council of Acoustical Consultants (NCAC) be engaged (see appendix 2).*

CALCULATING A-WEIGHTED SOUND LEVELS (dB_A)

1. Measure the octave band sound pressure levels at 125, 250, 500, 1000, 2000 and 4000 Hz with a sound level meter set on the flat or linear frequency weighting scale.

2. Apply the following correction numbers to the octave band levels to obtain equivalent levels for A-weighted octave band analysis:

Octave band center frequency, Hz	125	250	500	1000	2000	4000
correction factor	-16	-9	-3	0	+1	+1

3. Successively combine each octave band level with the next, using the following difference table:

If the difference in dB between two levels is:	0	1	2-3	5-7	8-9	10 or more
Add to the higher level:	3	2.5	2	1.5	0.5	0

4. Round the final answer to obtain the total dB_A level (Figure A3-1).

APPENDIX 3

How to calculate A weighted sound levels (dBA)

1. Measure the octave band sound pressure levels at 125, 250, 500, 1000, 2000 and 4000 Hz with a sound level meter set on the flat or linear frequency weighting scale.

2. Apply the following correction numbers to the octave band levels to obtain equivalent levels for A weighted octave band analysis.

Octave band center frequency, Hz	125	250	500	1000	2000	4000
Correction factor	-16	-9	-3	0	+1	+1

3. Successively combine each octave band level with the next, using the following difference table.

If the difference in dB between two levels is—	0	1	2-3	4	5-7	8-9	10 or more
Add to the higher level—	3	2.5	2	1.5	1	0.5	0

4. Round the final answer to obtain the total dBA level.

Example:

Frequency (Hz)	125	250	500	1000	2000	4000
Octave band level (dB)	108	103	99	104	101	85
Correction	-16	-9	-3	0	+1	+1
	92	94	96	104	102	86

+ 2 dB 96
+ 3 dB 99
+ 1 dB 105
+ 2 dB 107
+ 0 dB .... The result is 107 dBA.

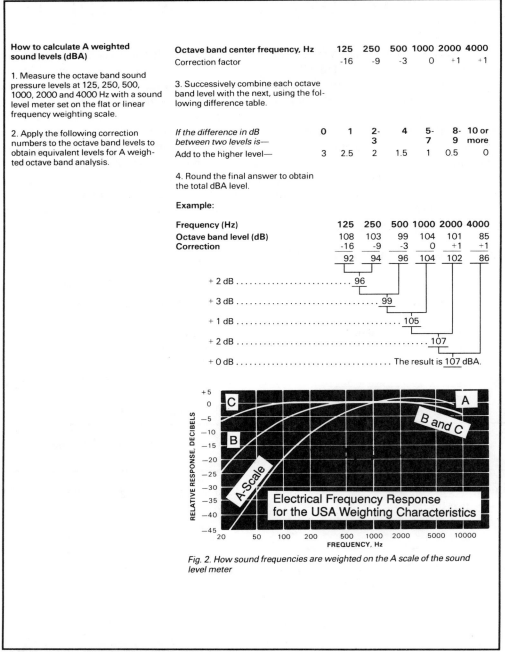

Fig. 2. How sound frequencies are weighted on the A scale of the sound level meter

Figure A3-1 - Example calculation of dB$_A$.

REVERBERANT SOUND CONTROL GUIDELINES

NCA members manufacture a wide range of products and materials that can be effectively employed to reduce excessive reverberant noise (i.e. reflected sounds that cause echoes). Two approaches may be used.

1. Where the overall steady state noise level must be reduced, control of the reverberant sound field itself is usually the best solution.

2. Where reverberant noise produces echoes in such spaces as arenas, gymnasiums, classrooms, factories and auditoriums, or where speech intelligibility from a public address system must be improved, control of the reverberation time is usually the best approach. Reverberation time is the interval required for a sound to decay 60 dB after it has been stopped. Generally this interval should be between 2.0 and 2.5 seconds in order to avoid echoes that interfere with speech intelligibility.

Most reverberant sound problems will involve a combination of these two approaches. For a thorough investigation of the acoustical environment that is to be treated, sound absorption coefficients should be considered at octave band center frequencies of 125, 250, 500, 1000, 2000 and 4000 Hz. Or, if a sound occurring at a particular frequency is known to be the major offender, calculations at that frequency alone may suffice. Also, a rough approximation of the solution to a reverberation noise or reverberation time problem may be accomplished using sound absorption characteristics of the environment at 500 Hz. When complex problems are encountered, NCA recommends engaging the services of an acoustical consultant who is a member of the National Council of Acoustical Consultants (NCAC).

The following procedure may be used for estimating the amount, type and array of acoustical control products necessary to control the reverberant noise problem:

1. Determine the existing sound absorption coefficients for the walls, floor and ceiling of the room or area to be treated. (See data tables in Appendix 4 for estimates if necessary.) This will establish baseline information for solving the reverberant noise problems.

2. Establish the acoustical design requirements for the room or area, considering such criteria as OSHA noise exposure limits or reverberation time desired.

3. Consult the data in Appendix 4, or manufacturer's published sound absorption coefficients and values for the products under consideration.

A worksheet for determining the reverberation time and amount of material required to be added to a room to achieve the desired reverberation time follows. A second worksheet with a specific example also follows.

Example:

Determine the change in the reverberant sound level and in the reverberation time at 500 Hz in a 200 by 100 by 30 foot room.
Ceiling: wood deck . . . . Sound absorption coefficient 0.14
Floor: concrete . . . . Sound absorption coefficient 0.01
Walls: gypsum
  wallboard . . . . Sound absorption coefficient 0.03

Acoustical treatment will consist of the following:
Suspended Fiberglas
  ceiling . . . . Sound absorption coefficient 0.90
¼" pile carpet
  on floor . . . . Sound absorption coefficient 0.15
Fiberglas nubby glass cloth board (on half the
  wall area) . . . . Sound absorption coefficient 0.73

The sabins of absorption in the room are calculated according to the following procedure:

	WALL	CEILING	FLOOR
UNTREATED ROOM			
1. List areas of room surfaces.	18,000	20,000	20,000
2. List sound absorption coefficient for each room surface.	.03	.14	.01
3. Multiply Line 2 by Line 1 to compute sabins.	540	2800	200
4. Add results on Line 3 for total sabins, all room surfaces.		3540	
5. List sabins for people in room.		—	
6. List sabins for space absorbers.		—	
7. Add Lines 4,5,6 to find total sabins for room.		3540	
ACOUSTICALLY TREATED ROOM —			
1. List areas of room surfaces.*	16,800*	20,000	20,000
2. List sound absorption coefficient for each room surface.	.03,.73	.90	.15
3. Multiply Line 2 by Line 1 to compute sabins, each half of walls	252+6132	18,000	3,000
4. Add results on Line 3 for total sabins, all room surfaces.		27,384	
5. List sabins for people in room.		—	
6. List sabins for space absorbers.		—	
7. Add Lines 4,5,6 to find total sabins for room.		27,384	

A To determine reduction in reverberant noise levels produced by adding sound absorbing material to a room use the following procedure:

1. Determine total sabins for untreated room.	3,540
2. Determine total sabins for room with added acoustical treatment.	27,384
3. Divide Line 2 by Line 1.	7.74
4. Take the logarithm of Line 3.	.89
5. Multiply Line 4 by 10 to obtain reduction in reverberant noise level. (Approximately 9 dB)	8.9 dB

To determine the change in reverberation time in the room described in this example after it has been acoustically treated as described, use the following procedure:

B UNTREATED ROOM

1. Calculate the volume of the room in cubic feet.	600,000
2. Multiply Line 1 by 0.05.	30,000
3. Determine total sabins for room.	3,540
4. Divide Line 2 by Line 3 for reverberation time in seconds.	8.47

B ACOUSTICALLY TREATED ROOM

1. Calculate the volume of the room in cubic feet.	560,000*
2. Multiply Line 1 by 0.05.	28,000
3. Determine total sabins for room.	27,384
4. Divide Line 2 by Line 3 for reverberation time in seconds.	1.02

The reduction of the reverberation time from 8.47 to 1.02 seconds will solve the reverberant sound problem very well.

Worksheet for solving reverberant sound problems

The sabins of absorption in a room are calculated according to the following procedure:

	WALL	CEILING	FLOOR
1. List areas of room surfaces.	_____	_____	_____
2. List sound absorption coefficient for each surface.	_____	_____	_____
3. Multiply Line 2 by Line 1 to compute sabins.	_____	_____	_____
4. Add results on Line 3 for total sabins, all room surfaces	_____		
5. List sabins for people in room.	_____		
6. List sabins for space absorbers.	_____		
7. Add Lines 4,5,6 to find total sabins for room.	_____		

A. To determine reduction in reverberant noise levels produced by adding sound absorbing material to a room, use the following procedure:

1. Determine total sabins for untreated room. _____
2. Determine total sabins for room with added acoustical treatment. _____
3. Divide Line 2 by Line 1. _____
4. Take the logarithm of Line 3. _____
5. Multiply Line 4 by 10 to obtain reduction in reverberant noise level. _____

The noise reduction in Line 5 can be improved successively by adding more sound absorbing material to the room and repeating Steps 2 through 5. The practical upper limit for reduction of reverberant noise levels is 10 to 12 dB. If estimates are in excess of this amount they should be carefully checked.

B. To determine the reverberation time in a room, use the following procedure:

1. Calculate the volume of the room in cubic feet. _____
2. Multiply Line 1 by 0.05. _____
3. Determine total sabins for room. _____
4. Divide Line 2 by Line 3 to obtain reverberation time, in seconds. _____

C. To determine the amount of sound absorbing material to be added to a room in order to achieve a desired reverberation time, use the following procedure:

1. Calculate the volume of the room in cubic feet. _____
2. Multiply Line 1 by 0.05. _____
3. List desired reverberation time in seconds. _____
4. Divide Line 2 by Line 3 for total sabins required in room. _____
5. Determine sabins for untreated room. _____
6. Subtract Line 5 from Line 4 for sabins of absorption to be added. _____

Additional sabins given on Line 6 will provide desired reverberation time. Select acoustical materials to provide this added absorption from the acoustical data

EXAMPLES OF SPR NOISE CONTROL

Example 1 - Controlling noise at its SOURCE

A large electric motor produces the noise levels shown in line 1 of the table at a nearby worker's station (Figure 3A-2).

Step 1(a):

A removable enclosure for the motor is to be built. To determine the approximate degree of noise reduction that can be expected, refer to the data tables in Appendix 4 (or manufacturer's data). Since 1/2" plywood is an economical and practical material with which to build an enclosure, we fill in the insertion loss values for a 1/2" plywood enclosure. These are shown on Line 2 in the table. (Data is from table II-3, Appendix 4.)

Subtracting these insertion loss values from the noise levels measured before acoustical treatment of the noise source, we find that the noise levels at the worker's station can be reduced by the enclosure to the levels shown in Line 3 of the table.

The 94 dB$_A$ sound level is determined by applying correction factors for the A weighted levels, and combining octave band levels, as was described in the previous section of this appendix. This level is still above OSHA allowances for exposure during an 8-hour day; in fact, a worker may only be subjected to this level for 4 hours. (See Figure 1-5.) The sound enclosure must be made more acoustically efficient.

Step 1(b):

Improving the sound attenuation may be accomplished by adding one inch thickness of medium density fiberglass insulation board to the **interior** surface of the 1/2" plywood enclosure. Similar results can be achieved with open cell foam readily available from NCA members. The increased insertion loss values are shown in Line 5 of the table. Subtracting these insertion loss values from Line 4, we find that the noise levels at the worker's station can be reduced to the levels shown in Line 6.

The 81 dB$_A$ sound level is well within OSHA allowances for 8-hour-day exposure. This example clearly shows the effectiveness of adding insulation board for source noise control. (Note: These results apply to an enclosure with no holes, seams or other sound leaks. If leaks exist, these insertion loss values will not be achieved.) If required, the inside surface of the enclosure could be covered with a plastic film to protect the insulation from oil or water vapor. However, such a film should not be more than one mill thick or it will have adverse acoustical effects.

Other solutions that address themselves to treating the source of noise might be to:

- Relocate the motor further from the worker's station.
- Replace the noisy motor with a quieter one.
- Check, and as required replace, worn gears or other moving parts which might be the underlying cause of the excessive noise.
- Consider active noise remedies.

Example 1 Step 1(a)	OCTAVE BAND CENTER FREQUENCIES, Hz						
	125	250	500	1000	2000	4000	dBA*
1. Noise level before treatment	108	103	99	104	101	85	107
2. Insertion loss, ½" plywood	-13	-11	-12	-12	-13	-15	
3. Noise level after treatment	95	92	87	92	88	70	94
Step 1(b)							
4. Noise level before treatment	108	103	99	104	101	85	107
5. Insertion loss, plywood + insulation	-18	-17	-23	-30	-38	-40	
6. Noise level after treatment	90	86	76	74	63	45	81
*See dBA calculation method.							

Figure A3-2 - Example 1 - SOURCE CONTROL

Controlling noise along its PATH

Sound, in traveling from a source to a listener, can take two paths. *One:* it may take a direct path, not striking any surface before arriving at the listener's location. *Two:* it may take an indirect path, being reflected from one or more surfaces. In most instances, both direct and indirect sound reaches the listeners position (Figure 3A-3).

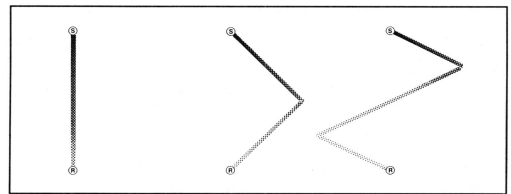

Figure A3-3 - Direct, single and multiple reflection sound paths from source to listener.

The most effective means of reducing indirect sound is to place sound absorptive materials on the surfaces the sound strikes. Thus, when the sound strikes these surfaces, most is absorbed and very little is reflected off the surface. Open cell foam and fiberglass are among the most efficient sound absorptive materials available. They can absorb up to 99% of the sound that strikes their surfaces. NCA members manufacture a wide range of products, from building insulation to acoustical ceiling panels, that can be used to absorb reflected sound. Where possible, the installation of an acoustical ceiling in a room or plant is one of the most effective means of reducing sound reflections. Various types and sizes of ceiling panels are available.

If the installation of a ceiling is not feasible because of the presence of pipes, lights, electrical wires, ducts or other systems, then unit sound absorbers (i.e. baffles) may be used in the ceiling area, or acoustical treatments may be applied to side walls or to the underside of the roof deck. As in the case of insulation for enclosures, a wide range of materials can be used for acoustical treatments depending on temperature, humidity, durability, density and surface finish requirements. If desired, these insulations can be covered by porous facings such as pegboard, expanded metal or cloth fabrics with little loss of sound absorption values. (See tables of sound absorption values in Appendix 4 or manufacturer's literature)

The worksheet provided earlier in this appendix can be used to estimate the reduction in reverberant noise level (or in reverberation time) that may be expected when sound absorbing materials are added to the space. Calculations should be done at each octave band to estimate the overall effect of treatment. How to use this work sheet is made clear in the accompanying example.

Direct sound cannot be reduced by the addition of sound-absorptive materials to surfaces, since by definition direct sound does not strike any surface before reaching the listener. The only effective means of reducing direct sound along its path is to install an acoustically effective barrier (i.e. a structure that is less than the full height and width of the noise path area) between the noise source and the receiver.

A sound barrier, to be most effective, must have two acoustical properties. *One:* the sound transmission loss or noise reduction capacity of the barrier must be high enough so that sound is attenuated in passing through the barrier. *Two:* it must be sound absorptive so that sound striking the barrier is absorbed and not reflected back into the area of the source. Since by definition a barrier is free-standing (i.e. it does not extend from the floor to the ceiling or roof), sound will be diffracted around the barrier in a similar manner to that in which light is diffracted around the corner of a building.

Depending on the size of the barrier, the location of the noise source and receiver relative to the barrier, and the frequency content of the noise source, the noise reduction across a barrier due to sound diffraction may approach 24 dB – the practical limit that can be expected of such measures. Therefore, it is imperative that the sound transmission loss of the barrier be at least 24 dB so sound doesn't pass through the barrier instead of being diffracted around it.

For most barriers, a septum with a weight of more than 1.5 lbs/sq. ft. (such as 1/2" plywood, 1/2" gypsum board, or 20 gauge sheet metal), plus at least two inches of fiberglass insulation on the source side of the barrier, should be sufficient. In some cases it may be necessary to construct a heavier barrier in order to reduce low frequency noise.

The nomogram in Figure A3-5, can be used to calculate the amount of sound attenuation in dB provided by a barrier blocking direct transmission of sound along a path from source to receiver. The barrier width should be twice its height to be effective.

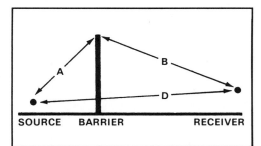

Figure A3-4 - Distances involved in determining barrier sound attenuation using nomogram in Figure A3-5.

In the nomogram, values for line (A + B − D) are determined by referring to Figure A3-4.

- Line A represents the distance from the noise source to the top of the barrier, in feet.
- Line B represents the distance from the receiver to the top of the barrier, in feet.
- Line D represents the straight line distance from the source to the receiver position, in feet.
- Line F of the nomogram (Figure A3-5) represents the octave band center frequency of the offending noise.

- The line at the right in Figure A3-5 labled dB, provides the attenuation in dB that is provided by the barrier.

Use of the nomogram is made clear in the following example.

Example 2 - Controlling noise along its PATH

The same motor, from example 1, is producing the same noise levels at the worker's station (see line 1 in Figure A3-6), but, for reasons of service accessibility, an enclosure is considered impractical. It is decided to treat the path of the noise by building a barrier between the motor and the worker's station adjacent to the motor location. Noise paths have been studied and it has been determined there is a good likelihood that reflected sound is not presenting a problem. (i.e. walls and ceilings have absorption coefficients of 0.85 or better). Distance D from the motor to the worker's ear is 10.4 feet; distance A from the motor to the top of the barrier is 6.4 feet; distance B from the worker's ear to the top of the barrier is 5.1

feet. The value (A + B - D) is determined to be 1.1 (see position 1 in Figure A3-7), and this value is located on the left hand line of the nomogram in Figure A3-5. Lines are drawn from this point through the octave band center frequency values on the middle line of the nomogram and extended to cross the right hand line, where barrier attenuation values in dB may be read for each frequency and entered in the calculations (Line 2 in Example 2, Figure A3-7). Subtracting these values from the octave band noise levels given in Example 1 and correcting for A scale weighting (per Figure A3-1), the overall result is 91 dB$_A$. This level exceeds OSHA allowances for 8-hour exposure, so the barrier nomogram is now used to determine the effect of placing the barrier closer to the noise source. When located one foot from the source, distance A becomes 4.1 feet and distance B is 9.1 feet. (distance D remains 10.4 feet.) The value (A + B - D) is now 2.8 (see position 2 in Figure 3A-6). Using the nomogram, barrier attenuation values are read on

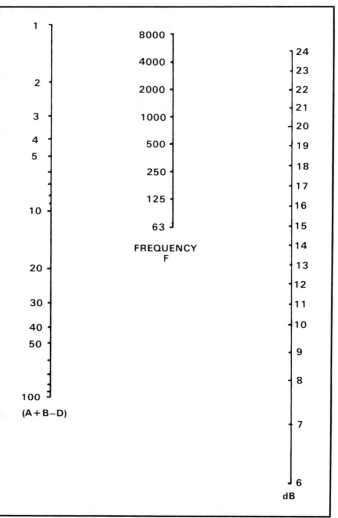

Figure A3-5 - Nomogram for determining barrier sound attenuation in dB.

Line 5 in Example 2 (Figure 3A-7). When motor noise levels are attenuated by these amounts to the levels on Line 6 in Example 2 and corrected for A scale weightings, the level becomes 88 dB$_A$, a level which is within OSHA exposure limits for an 8-hour day.

The nomogram can be used in this manner to optimize barrier height given a fixed location, or to optimize its location given a fixed height.

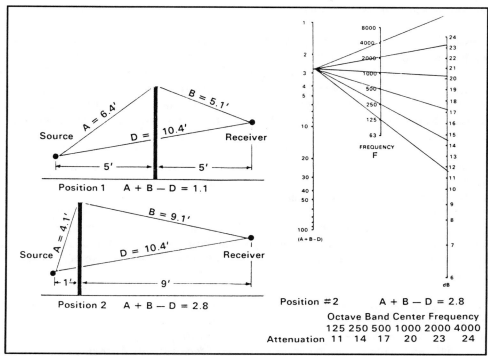

Figure A3-6 - Example 2, barrier attenuation schematic and nomogram.

Example 2 Step 1(a)	OCTAVE BAND CENTER FREQUENCIES, Hz						
	125	250	500	1000	2000	4000	dBA*
1. Noise level before treatment	108	103	99	104	101	85	107
2. Barrier attenuation, location 1	-9	-11	-13	-16	-19	-22	
3. Noise level after treatment	99	92	86	88	82	63	91
Step 1(b)							
4. Noise level before treatment	108	103	99	104	101	85	107
5. Barrier attenuation, location 2	-11	-14	-17	-20	-23	-24	
6. Noise level after treatment	97	89	82	84	78	61	88
*See dBA calculation method.							

Figure A3-7 - Example 2, barrier attenuation calculation

The above result applies to a condition where no reflected sound reaches the worker's station. If there is any reflected sound, these transmission loss values will not be achieved unless adjacent reflecting surfaces -- walls, ceiling, or other equipment in the area -- are also acoustically treated.

Controlling Noise at the RECEIVER

The most commonly used measures for receiver noise control are ear plugs or ear protectors. These, however, are classified by OSHA as **"temporary measurers."** OSHA requires **"permanent solutions"** known as Engineering or Management Controls. And, the only permanent methods of reducing noise at the receiver position is to build a partial or complete enclosure around the receiver/listener or utilize active noise measures. The latter is considered elsewhere in this manual. An enclosure for a listener is very similar to an enclosure for a noise source.

The basic difference between the two is that an employee enclosure must provide an environment in which the employee can function efficiently and comfortably. This usually means that lights, windows, a door, and a ventilation system must be provided. These may degrade the overall acoustical performance of the enclosure due to sound leaks and lower noise reduction values of doors and windows. (See last section of Appendix 3 for a technique to estimate the STC of a composite structure.) Therefore, greater emphasis must be placed on details of designing and building an employee enclosure than in the case of a noise source enclosure.

The use of resilient furring channels on wood studs or 25 gage drywall steel studs, with gypsum wallboard with a core of soft fibrous insulation, plus liberal use of caulking to seal sound leaks, is an excellent start in the design of a worker enclosure. In many instances, controls, dials and gauges may be installed in the enclosure to further reduce the time necessary for the employee to spend outside it in the noisy environment. Doors and windows should, if possible, be located on the side away from the noise source, and provision for ventilation should be located and constructed so the system will not conduct noise into the enclosure.

Example 3 - Controlling noise at the RECEIVER

The same motor is producing the same noise levels at the worker's station (line 1 in Figure A3-8). A motor enclosure is impractical; the path of sound reaching the worker's station is such that a barrier or partition will not block sufficient sound. Therefore, the worker's station needs to be enclosed.

The effective noise reduction that will be achieved at the worker's station due to the introduction of a total enclosure is the sum of two factors: the sound transmission loss of the enclosure boundaries, plus a room adjustment factor which is equal to ten times the logarithm of the ratio of the room sound absorption to the total surface area of the noise-exposed room boundaries.

Step 1(a):
For the purposes of this example we will assume that the room adjustment factor is given in Lines 2 and 6 of the table. Referring to Appendix 4 of this manual, we find the Sound

Example 3 Step 1(a)	OCTAVE BAND CENTER FREQUENCIES, Hz						
	125	250	500	1000	2000	4000	dBA*
1. Noise level without enclosure	108	103	99	104	101	85	107
2. Room adjustment factors	-0	-1	-3	-4	-4	-4	
3. Transmission loss, plain wall	-16	-23	-37	-45	-46	-37	
4. Noise level within enclosure	92	79	59	55	51	44	77
Step 1(b)							
5. Noise level without enclosure	108	103	99	104	101	85	107
6. Room adjustment factors	-0	-1	-3	-4	-4	-4	
7. Transmission loss, insulated wall	-24	-35	-47	-54	-57	-42	
8. Noise level within enclosure	84	67	49	46	40	39	68
*See dBA calculation method.							

Figure A3-8 - Example 3, Controlling Noise at RECEIVER

Transmission Loss values for a wall constructed of 3-5/8" metal studs with 1/2" gypsum board on both sides. These are listed on Line 3 of the table. While the resulting 77 dB$_A$ sound level inside the enclosure (line 4) is within OSHA noise exposure limits for an 8-hour day as shown in Figure 1-5, it is still considered uncomfortably noisy. Therefore, it is decided to add acoustical treatment to the enclosure.

Step 1(b):
Adding 3-1/2" of fiberglass building insulation to the stud cavity of the enclosure will provide additional sound transmission loss. The total transmission loss (metal stud and gypsum board wall plus building insulation), also taken from Appendix 4 of this manual, is listed on Line 7 in the table. Subtracting the total effective noise reduction values from the noise levels before treatment, we find the noise level within the worker's enclosure can be reduced to 68 dB$_A$ (see values on Line 8 of Figure A3-8).

The calculated dB$_A$ reading is well within OSHA exposure limits. It can also be expected to result in a noise level within the enclosure approximating that of a normal, moderately noisy shop. The results apply to an enclosure without sound leaks, without a plate glass window facing the noise source, with an acoustically rated door also facing away from the noise source, and with all ventilation and other openings properly treated to avoid sound leaks. If leaks exist, these sound transmission loss values will not be achieved.

CONTROLLING ENVIRONMENTAL NOISE

Keeping outside noises out

Measuring sound transmission loss and sound absorption coefficients of building materials provides a means of predicting the noise level within a space. The noise in a given space may come from a source in that space or from an adjacent space. This section will deal with noise sources outside a building.

Determining the influence of outside sources

Use the following equation to predict the noise level in a room exposed to an outside noise source:

$$L_p(\text{int}) = L_p(\text{ext}) - TL + 10 \log S/A + ADJ$$

$L_p(\text{int}) =$ Predicted average sound pressure level in the building interior at a given frequency in dB

$L_p(\text{ext}) =$ measured or predicted average sound pressure level at the building exterior for a given frequency band, in dB

$TL =$ sound transmission loss of the exterior wall or roof at a given frequency band, in dB

$S =$ total exposed exterior surface area of room, in sq. ft.

$A =$ total sabins of absorption in the room at a given frequency band

$ADJ =$ adjustment factor which takes into consideration certain characteristics of the sound source. Example: for aircraft traverses or for continuous traffic, the sound field incident on the building facade is a reasonable approximation to the reverberant field condition in which the TL values were measured. For such a case, the term $ADJ = 3$ dB.

The term ADJ is equal to 3 dB only when the sound field incident on the facade approximates a reverberant field condition. When this is not the case, the term ADJ takes a more general form. Thus, $ADJ = 3$ dB $+ G$ where G, stated in dB is an adjustment for the geometrical arrangement of the noise source relative to the building facade. The sound transmission loss of a building component is dependent on the angle of incidence of the sound wave striking the component. Since TL is determined with random incidence sound, adjustments must be made for situations where the sound is incident from fixed angles such as from a stationary source. Figure A3-9 shows values for G to be used for different angles of incidence relative to the building facade.

DETERMINING THE SOUND TRANSMISSION LOSS OF A COMPOSITE PARTITION

A partition may have different components, such as doors or windows. The designer needs to know the transmission loss of this composite partition before the overall noise reduction can be calculated.

Angle of incidence, degrees	Adjustment G, dB
0 – 30	-3
30 – 60	-1
Random	0
60 – 80	+2
Greater than 80	+5

Figure A3-9 - Adjustment G to allow for primary angles of incidence

Design considerations

The equation for predicting the noise level in a building interior can be used in two ways. *One:* if a preliminary exterior wall design exists, the interior noise level can be predicted for that design and compared to code compliance criteria. *Two:* if a preliminary design does not exist, the minimum required sound transmission loss required to meet code requirements can be determined without first determining construction details.

To screen proposed facade constructions, or any other partition system, a simplified equation for predicting interior noise levels uses the STC value of a construction in place of transmission loss (TL) values. In addition, other noise level descriptors such as A-weighted dB levels (dB_A), day-night average level (L_{dn}), or community noise equivalent level (CNEL) may be used for the exterior noise levels $L_p(ext)$ in the equation. This equation is thus written as follows:

$$L(int) = L(ext) - STC + 10 \log S/A + ADJ$$

- $L(int)$ = approximate interior noise level in the same unit as used for L(ext)
- $L(ext)$ = approximate exterior noise level in dB, dB_A, L_{dn} or CNEL
- STC = Sound Transmission Class of the exterior facade construction
- ADJ = 3 + G + F, where G = values in Figure A3-8. F = adjustment for frequency spectrum characteristics of the noise source (Figure A3-10).

The factor 10 log S/A can be approximated using Figure A3-11 to determine the value A and the chart shown in Figure A3-12 to determine log S/A.

The above method is only an approximation and should be used only as a screening tool. Engineering calculations for code compliance may necessitate the services of an acoustical consultant.

The first method is most useful when the designer has a particular construction in mind. It will determine easily whether a particular design will work acoustically by first determining

134 APPENDIX 3

Noise source	Adjustment F, dB
Jet aircraft within 500 feet	0
Train wheel/rail noise	2
Road traffic, few trucks	4
Jet aircraft at 3000 feet	5
Road traffic, over 10% trucks	6
Diesel-electric locomotive	6

Figure A3-10 - Adjustment F to allow for spectrum shape of common outdoor noise sources

the composite STC of the exterior wall based on the individual STC values and surface area of each element of the composite wall.

The composite STC can be estimated with the use of Figure A3-12 as follows (assuming two elements of the composite):

First: calculate the difference between the STC of the two elements (see Appendix 4 for exterior wall, door and window values).

Second: calculate the area percentage of the lower STC element.

Third: Determine the adjustment to be

	Types of furnishings			
	HARD: sound reflective walls, floor and ceiling, no drapes	STANDARD: reflective walls, acoustical ceiling, hard floor	SOFT: acoustical ceiling, carpet or drapes	VERY SOFT: acoustical ceiling, carpet or drapes and wall furniture
"A" factor	0.3	0.8	0.9	1.0

Figure A3-11 - "A" factors for estimating room absorption from floor area

subtracted from the higher STC value to give the composite STC of the two elements.

Fourth: Repeat the procedure for additional elements in the composite construction.

Substitution of the values into the facade equation given above will give a prediction of the interior noise level. If lower than design criteria values, the design is acceptable.

Comparison of individual noise contributions indicates which element is the weak link. This component can either be changed in size or in type to reduce its contribution. Optimized design calls for each wall component to be designed so as to contribute equally to solving the problem. However, this usually impractical for reasons of material or architectural design.

Example: Assume a stucco wall with insulation resilient channel construction. Appendix 4 lists an STC of 57 for such a design. The wall has a solid wood door in it. Appendix 4 lists an STC of 27 for the door. The door area is 13% of the total wall area.

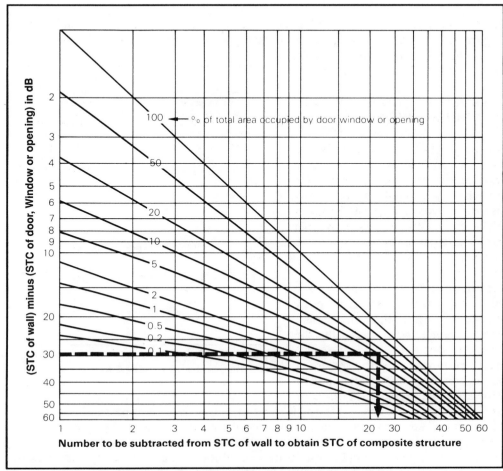

Figure A3-12 - Chart for determining STC of a composite structure

To find the composite STC: 57 - 27 = 30. Find this STC difference (30) on the vertical axis of Figure A3-12 and move horizontally to 13%, the door area. Drop to the horizontal axis to read the number to be subtracted from the wall STC. Thus 57 - 23 = 34.

CONTROLLING NOISE WITHIN PLANT BOUNDARIES:

With the passage of federal, state and local noise ordinances, it is becoming more important that objectionable noise be prevented from being transmitted beyond adjacent property boundaries. This is especially true where residential areas are adjacent to plants.

There are several ways to contain noise within the boundaries of a noisy industrial operation. First, one should attempt to quiet the source using the techniques discussed under source control. Be sure to include purchase of quiet equipment, and active and/or passive noise suppressors (mufflers or noise canceling) in the design effort. If these measures have been pursued extensively and other measures are required, consider locating the noise producing equipment within the central zone of the plant or building. Another way to contain sound is to use exterior building shells with high sound transmission loss values. Be sure to include consideration of sound leaks and flanking paths as discussed in the sections dealing with reducing noise along the path. Where vents and ducts are transmitting the source, consider lining the inside of the ducts with sound absorbing materials or installing duct attenuators. If a fence is to be constructed, utilize the principals outlined in an earlier section for barriers. Where specific sound sources can be defined as the intrusive noise, consider active noise treatment measures.

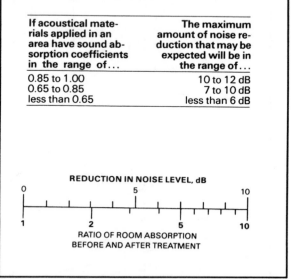

Figure A3-13 - Noise reduction when sound absorbing material is added to a room

If acoustical materials applied in an area have sound absorption coefficients in the range of...	The maximum amount of noise reduction that may be expected will be in the range of...
0.85 to 1.00	10 to 12 dB
0.65 to 0.85	7 to 10 dB
less than 0.65	less than 6 dB

CONTROLLING NOISE IN ADJACENT OFFICE AREAS

Disconcertingly high noise levels are often encountered in office areas adjacent to noisy industrial operations. Even though such noise levels may not approach the exposure limits established by OSHA for an 8-hour day, they may be of sufficient intensity to distract and annoy office occupants, interfering with efficiency and making speech communication difficult.

In fact, noise levels of 55 to 60 dB_A are generally considered excessive for the office environment.

Chapter 8 provides an extensive discussion of the measures that may be taken to provide speech privacy between work stations. Background masking sound, provided it is not so high that it is in and of itself intrusive, has been effective in controlling some exterior noise. When the intrusive noise is greater than 55 dB_A, other measures should be employed. Identification of the specific source and implementing appropriate controls is the most effective. If quieting the source is not practical, then the barrier must be sufficient to block the intrusive noise. Design the partitions to have an effective STC and eliminate all sound leaks and flanking paths.

For a comprehensive discussion of office acoustics, refer to Chapter 2 of the book *Planning and Designing the Office Environment, Second Edition*, Harris, D. A. et. al., Van Nostrand Reinhold, New York, NY, 1990.

NOISE REDUCTION WITHIN A ROOM

The amount of noise reduction obtained in a confined area, such as a conference room, auditorium, classroom, lunch room, natatorium, meeting rooms, or sanctuary, by adding sound absorbing materials, depends on several factors. The size and geometry of the room, the sound absorbing properties of existing materials, the location of the noise sources, the amount of sound absorbing material added in the space, and the placement of such material are factors to consider. It is therefore impossible to determine precisely the degree of noise reduction that can be expected from acoustical treatments in such a space without taking into account the above factors. An experienced acoustician or member of the National Council of Acoustical Consultants (NCAC), trained in solving noise control problems, should be able to consider these factors and arrive at fairly accurate calculations of the effectiveness of noise control measures. While any noise control measure must be considered as a unique case, with effectiveness varying from case to case, the information in figure A3-13 can be regarded as a general guide.

COMMUNITY NOISE AND OTHER NOISE

Noise from freeways, airports, and other community supported sources or events are the focus of considerable attention in our society. These issues are complex both from a technical and social standpoint. The legal implications of these noise problems are beyond the scope of this manual. Where specific noise sources are identifiable and a solution that involves the Source, Path, and Receiver (as discussed within this manual) are to be implemented, those techniques are applicable. While several volumes have been produced on community noise there is not yet general agreement in the acoustical community. For more information, it is recommended that the reader contact the officers and members of ASTM Committee E-33.08 on Community Noise. Local communities have implemented noise regulations of many types. Some are the typical "barking dog" variety, while others have implemented specific limits of sound level from a source at a specific distance. An example is Redondo Beach, CA, where the so called "boom boxes" (loud vehicle music amplifiers) are limited to a specific sound level meter reading at a specified distance from the vehicle. While measures discussed in this manual may be utilized, these regulations are primarily designed to encourage the operator to *control the source using management controls.*

Design of freeway noise barriers and the like is akin to, but more complex than, design of part-high barriers discussed earlier. Where the noise situation does not clearly fall in one of the sections discussed earlier, namely the Source, Path and Receiver controls, NCA recommends it be addressed by a member in good standing of the National Council of Acoustical Consultants. Additional information may be obtained from the author by calling 213 377-9958. A whole technology has evolved for the prediction of highway noise including several computer programs based on traffic volume, type of vehicles by percent, # of traffic lanes and the incline or grade.

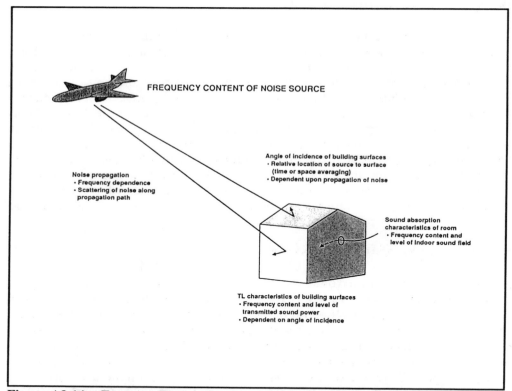

Figure A3-14 - Factors affecting the A-weighted noise level reduction of a building envelope for aircraft flyovers.

Similarly, a whole technology exists for airport noise. Again, this is a specialized field complete with computer simulations and a whole new set of terms specific to the circumstances. Contact the author or the Federal Aviation Authority (FAA) for additional information. Factors affecting the A-weighted noise level reduction of a typical building envelope are shown in Figure A3-14. Figure A3-15 shows typical noise intrusion paths.

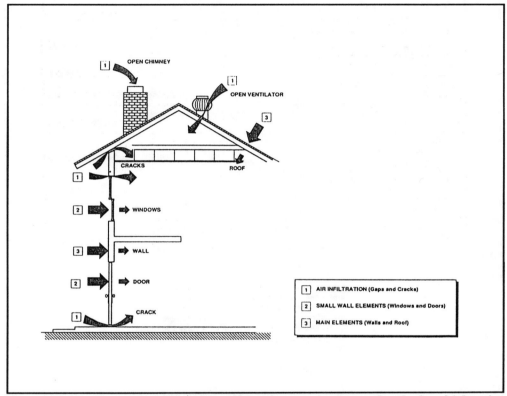

Figure A3-15 - Conceptual illustration of the three major types of paths by which noise is transmitted to building interiors.

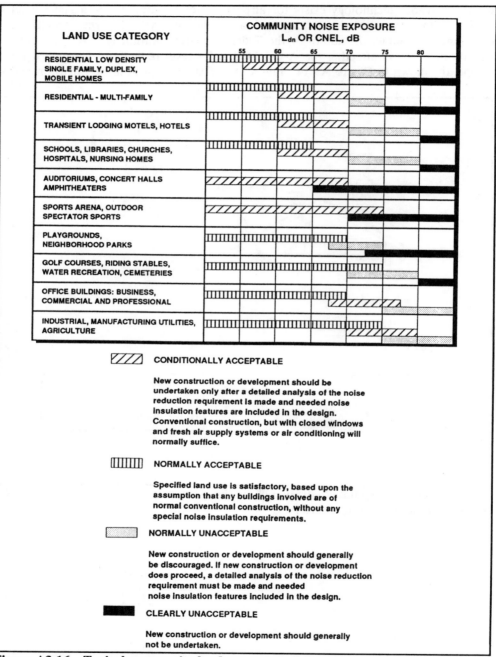

Figure A3-16 - Typical community land use compatibility

Appendix 4 - ACOUSTICAL DATA

Section 1 - SOUND ABSORBING MATERIALS

The data in these tables have been organized by type of product. Unless otherwise noted, the tests were conducted in a NVLAP approved facility in accordance with ASTM C 423, Standard Test Method for Sound Absorption and Sound Absorption Coefficients by the Reverberation Room Method. Sound absorption coefficients for each sample were measured over one-third-octave bands and are reported at the preferred octave band center frequencies. In some cases, the measured sound absorption coefficients are greater than 1.00. As recommended by the test method, these values are reported as measured and not adjusted. The corresponding NRC for a material may also be greater than 1.00 according to the ASTM test method. The sound absorption coefficients of these materials are not significantly affected by coverings such as expanded sheet metal, metal lath, hardware cloth, screening or glass cloth. When other coverings having less open surfaces are used, the description so notes the material. **For additional information, consult Noise Control Association Manufacturers Technical Literature.**

Notes to sound absorption tables:

(1) Mounting (see Figure 2-6 and ASTM E795 for additional details):

- Type A (formerly #4) - Material placed against a solid backing such as a block wall.
- Mod. 7 - Material placed against 24 gauge sheet metal over a 16 inch air space. This mounting configuration is typical of a sheet metal enclosure with insulation on one side. Data include facings exposed to sound source, if specified.
- E-405 (formerly #7) - Material placed over a 16 inch air space. Data include facings exposed to sound source if specified. This mounting simulates a typical suspended ceiling system in a commercial building.
- No. 6 - Material placed over 24 gauge galvanized sheet metal with 1 inch air space.

(2) Facings:

- FRK (Foil Reinforced Kraft): Foil faced laminate with glass fiber reinforcing and kraft backing.
- ASJ (All Service Jacket): An embossed laminate of white kraft facing with glass fiber reinforcing and a foil backing.

NRC - Noise Reduction Coefficient

Product Type & Thickness		Mounting (1)	OCTAVE BAND CENTER FREQUENCIES, Hz						
			125	250	500	1000	2000	4000	NRC
3.50"	(R-11), insulation exposed to sound	A	.34	.85	1.09	.97	.97	1.12	.95
6.25"	(R-19), insulation exposed to sound	A	.64	1.14	1.09	.99	1.00	1.21	1.05
3.50"	(R-11), insulation exposed to sound	E-405	.80	.98	1.01	1.04	.98	1.15	1.00
6.25"	(R-19), insulation exposed to sound	E-405	.86	1.03	1.13	1.02	1.04	1.13	1.05
3.50"	(R-11), FRK facing exposed to sound	A	.56	1.11	1.16	.61	.40	.21	.80
6.25"	(R-19), FRK facing exposed to sound	A	.94	1.33	1.02	.71	.56	.39	.90

Table I-1. Sound absorption coefficients of 0.5 lb. density fiberglass building insulation

Product Type & Thickness		Mounting (1)	OCTAVE BAND CENTER FREQUENCIES, Hz						
			125	250	500	1000	2000	4000	NRC
2.5"	(R-8)	A	.21	.62	.93	.92	.91	1.03	.85
3.5"	(R-11)	A	.38	.88	1.13	1.03	.97	1.12	1.00
2.5"	(R-8)	E-405	.59	.84	.79	.94	.96	1.12	.90
3.5"	(R-11)	E-405	.73	.98	.98	1.05	1.08	1.15	1.00

Table I-2, *Sound absorption coefficients of 0.8 lb. density fiberglass insulation batts.*

Product Type & Thickness	Mounting (1)	125	250	500	1000	2000	4000	NRC
1, plain, 1" thick	A	.17	.33	.64	.83	.90	.92	.70
1, plain, 2" thick	A	.22	.67	.98	1.02	.98	1.00	.90
1, plain, 3" thick	A	.43	1.17	1.26	1.09	1.03	1.04	1.15
1, plain, 4" thick	A	.73	1.29	1.22	1.06	1.00	.97	1.15
1, plain, 1" thick	Mod. 7	.38	.34	.68	.82	.87	.96	.70
1, plain, 2" thick	Mod. 7	.44	.66	1.07	1.06	.99	1.06	.95
1, plain, 3" thick	Mod. 7	.53	.96	1.19	1.07	1.05	1.03	1.05
1, plain, 4" thick	Mod. 7	.61	1.10	1.20	1.11	1.08	1.09	1.10
1, plain, 1" thick	E-405	.32	.41	.70	.83	.93	1.02	.70
1, plain, 2" thick	E-405	.44	.68	1.00	1.09	1.06	1.10	.95
1, plain, 3" thick	E-405	.77	1.08	1.16	1.09	1.05	1.18	1.10
1, plain, 4" thick	E-405	.87	1.14	1.24	1.17	1.18	1.28	1.20
3, plain, 1" thick	A	.11	.28	.68	.90	.93	.96	.70
3, plain, 2" thick	A	.17	.86	1.14	1.07	1.02	.98	1.00
3, plain, 3" thick	A	.53	1.19	1.21	1.08	1.01	1.04	1.10
3, plain, 4" thick	A	.84	1.24	1.24	1.08	1.00	.97	1.15
3, plain, 1" thick	Mod. 7	.33	.28	.62	.88	.96	1.04	.70
3, plain, 2" thick	Mod. 7	.38	.63	1.10	1.07	1.05	1.05	.95
3, plain, 3" thick	Mod. 7	.45	.98	1.17	1.06	1.00	1.02	1.05
3, plain, 4" thick	Mod. 7	.62	1.10	1.15	1.05	.99	1.01	1.05
3, plain, 1" thick	E-405	.32	.32	.73	.93	1.01	1.10	.75
3, plain, 2" thick	E-405	.40	.73	1.14	1.13	1.06	1.10	1.00
3, plain, 3" thick	E-405	.66	.93	1.13	1.10	1.11	1.14	1.05
3, plain, 4" thick	E-405	.65	1.01	1.20	1.14	1.10	1.16	1.10
5, plain, 1" thick	A	.02	.27	.63	.85	.93	.95	.65
5, plain, 2" thick	A	.16	.71	1.02	1.01	.99	.99	.95
5, plain, 3" thick	A	.54	1.12	1.23	1.07	1.01	1.05	1.10
5, plain, 4" thick	A	.75	1.19	1.17	1.05	.97	.98	1.10
5, plain, 1" thick	Mod. 7	.32	.30	.66	.90	.95	1.01	.70
5, plain, 2" thick	Mod. 7	.39	.59	1.06	1.08	1.05	1.13	.95
5, plain, 3" thick	Mod. 7	.49	.93	1.15	1.06	.99	1.00	1.05
5, plain, 4" thick	Mod. 7	.57	1.06	1.13	1.02	.94	1.00	1.05
5, plain, 1" thick	E-405	.30	.34	.68	.87	.97	1.06	.70
5, plain, 2" thick	E-405	.39	.63	1.06	1.13	1.09	1.10	1.00
5, plain, 3" thick	E-405	.66	.92	1.11	1.12	1.10	1.19	1.05
5, plain, 4" thick	E-405	.59	.91	1.15	1.11	1.11	1.19	1.10
3, FRK faced, 1" thick (2)	A	.18	.75	.58	.72	.62	.35	.65
3, FRK faced, 2" thick	A	.63	.56	.95	.74	.60	.35	.75
3, FRK faced, 1" thick	Mod. 7	.31	.45	.62	.65	.51	.28	.55
3, FRK faced, 2" thick	Mod. 7	.38	.51	.83	.73	.53	.37	.65
3, FRK faced, 1" thick	E-405	.33	.49	.62	.78	.66	.45	.65
3, FRK faced, 2" thick	E-405	.45	.47	.97	.93	.65	.42	.75

Table I-3. Sound absorption coefficients of fiberglass boards. 1 = 1 lb. density, 3 = 3 lb. density, 5 = 5 lb. density (nominal).

Product Type & Thickness	Mounting (1)	OCTAVE BAND CENTER FREQUENCIES, Hz						
		125	250	500	1000	2000	4000	NRC
5, FRK faced, 1" thick	A	.27	.66	.33	.66	.51	.41	.55
5, FRK faced, 2" thick	A	.60	.50	.63	.82	.45	.34	.60
5, FRK faced, 1" thick	Mod. 7	.25	.48	.28	.57	.39	.30	.45
5, FRK faced, 2" thick	Mod. 7	.38	.36	.39	.37	.56	.38	.40
5, FRK faced, 1" thick	E-405	.29	.52	.33	.72	.58	.53	.55
5, FRK faced, 2" thick	E-405	.50	.36	.70	.90	.52	.47	.60
3, ASJ faced, 1" thick (3)	A	.17	.71	.59	.68	.54	.30	.65
3, ASJ faced, 2" thick	A	.47	.62	1.01	.81	.51	.32	.75
3, ASJ faced, 1" thick	E-405	.27	.54	.57	.66	.58	.36	.60
3, ASJ faced, 2" thick	E-405	.53	.44	.93	.77	.55	.35	.65
5, ASJ faced, 1" thick	A	.20	.64	.33	.56	.54	.33	.50
5, ASJ faced, 2" thick	A	.58	.49	.73	.76	.55	.35	.65
5, ASJ faced, 1" thick	E-405	.24	.58	.29	.75	.57	.41	.55
5, ASJ faced, 2" thick	E-405	.42	.35	.69	.80	.55	.42	.60

Table I-4. Sound absorption coefficients of faced fiberglass insulation boards. Facing exposed to sound.

Product Type & Thickness	Mounting (1)	OCTAVE BAND CENTER FREQUENCIES, Hz						
		125	250	500	1000	2000	4000	NRC
MBI, vinyl facing, 2" thick	A	.21	.63	1.10	.74	.33	.17	.70
MBI, vinyl facing, 3" thick	A	.38	.98	1.20	.62	.42	.24	.80
MBI, vinyl facing, 4" thick	A	.56	1.22	1.08	.64	.48	.23	.85
MBI, 1 mil Tedlar facing, 5"	A	.83	1.35	1.06	.85	.76	.54	1.00

Table I-5. Sound absorption coefficients of fiberglass metal building insulation.

Product Type & Thickness	Mounting (1)	OCTAVE BAND CENTER FREQUENCIES, Hz						
		125	250	500	1000	2000	4000	NRC
1" thick, economy	A	.04	.24	.70	.98	.99	.95	.75
1" thick, deluxe	A	.08	.37	.84	.99	1.01	1.02	.75

Table I-6. Sound absorption coefficients of fiberglass roof form board.

Product Type & Thickness	Mounting (1)	125	250	500	1000	2000	4000	NRC
1"	F-25	.34	.52	.73	.96	1.10	1.09	.85
1½"	No. 6	.25	.72	1.05	1.04	1.02	1.08	.95
2"	No. 6	.31	.81	1.16	1.09	1.06	1.13	1.05

Table I-7. Sound absorption coefficients of fiberglass duct liner board.

Product Type & Thickness	Mounting	125	250	500	1000	2000	4000
3"x24"x48" panel made with 2 layers of 1.5" 4.5 pcf glass fiber board covered with ½ oz./sq. yd. ripstop nylon	Major axis vertical with 6" spacing between units, 3" distance from mounting surface	2.8	8.6	17.2	17.8	16.0	11.7
3"x24"x48" panel made with 2 layers of 1.5" 4.5 pcf glass fiber board covered with glass cloth facing	Major axis horizontal with 6" spacing between units, 5¼" distance from mounting surface	3.4	8.2	16.6	18.0	18.8	19.2
3"x12"x48" panel made with 2 layers of 1.5" 4.5 pcf glass fiber board covered with ½ oz./sq. yd. ripstop nylon	Single unit with axis horizontal, 5¼" distance from mounting surface	0.7	5.3	10.3	11.6	10.2	7.5
12"x12"x48" rectangular prism made with 1.5", 4.5 pcf glass fiber board covered with ½ oz./sq. yd. ripstop nylon	Major axis vertical with 48" spacing between units, placed on mounting surface	3.6	10.4	15.2	17.4	15.6	11.5
12"x12"x48" triangular prism made with 1.5", 4.5 pcf glass fiber board covered with ½ oz./sq. yd. ripstop nylon	Major axis horizontal with 6" spacing between units, 32" distance from mounting surface	4.4	10.6	15.2	17.6	15.9	12.0
6" I.D., 9" O.D. glass fiber pipe insulation 36" long, covered with ½ oz./sq. yd. ripstop nylon	Major axis horizontal with 6" spacing between units, 36.5" distance from mounting surface	2.0	4.2	6.4	7.0	7.8	5.4

Table I-8. Sound absorption values, Sabines/Unit for miscellaneous space sound absorbers.

Product Type & Thickness	Mounting (1)	125	250	500	1000	2000	4000	NRC
Shasta, 5/8" film faced	E-405	.76	.71	.60	.76	.79	.74	.70
Shasta, 3/4" film faced	E-405	.72	.84	.70	.79	.76	.81	.75
Shasta, 1" film faced	E-405	.76	.84	.72	.89	.85	.81	.85
Random Fissured, 5/8" film faced	E-405	.66	.76	.60	.80	.89	.80	.75
Random Fissured, 3/4" film faced	E-405	.68	.81	.68	.78	.85	.80	.80
Random Fissured, 1" film faced	E-405	.74	.85	.68	.86	.90	.79	.80
Stonebrooke, 1" film faced	E-405	.56	.63	.69	.83	.71	.55	.70
Stonebrooke, 2" film faced	E-405	.52	.82	.88	.91	.75	.55	.85
Stonebrooke, 3" film faced	E-405	.64	.88	1.02	.91	.84	.62	.90
Milano, 5/8", painted mineral board	E-405	.25	.34	.41	.56	.65	.63	.50

Table I-9, Sound absorption coefficients of film faced fiberglass and painted mineral ceiling boards.

Product Type & Thickness	Mounting (1)	125	250	500	1000	2000	4000	NRC
Nubby, 3/4"	E-405	.81	.94	.65	.87	1.00	.96	.85
Nubby, 1"	E-405	.78	.92	.79	1.00	1.03	1.10	.95
Nubby, 1 1/2"	E-405	.80	.96	.88	1.04	1.05	1.06	1.00
Omega, 3/4"	E-405	.63	.87	.68	.92	1.00	1.12	.85
Omega, 1"	E-405	.71	.89	.76	.98	.98	1.06	.90
Omega, 1 1/2"	E-405	.80	.99	.87	1.05	1.04	1.08	1.00
Nubby Perfect, 2"	E-405	.53	.87	.99	1.10	1.05	1.01	1.00

Table I-10, Sound absorption coefficients of fiberglass, glass cloth faced acoustical ceiling panels.

Product Type & Thickness	Mounting (1)	125	250	500	1000	2000	4000	NRC
Wrapped edge	A	.04	.29	.76	1.03	1.05	1.08	.80
Monolithic	A	.05	.30	.80	1.00	1.02	.95	.80
Nubby glass cloth	A	.07	.27	.64	.92	1.03	.97	.70

Table I-11, Sound absorption coefficients of fiberglass needle punched faced wall treatments.

Product Type & Thickness		OCTAVE BAND CENTER FREQUENCIES, Hz						
		125	250	500	1000	2000	4000	NRC
3, 1" thick, unfaced	(1)	.06	.20	.68	.91	.96	.95	.70
3, 1" thick + ¼" pegboard	(2)	.08	.32	1.13	.76	.34	.12	.65
3, 1" thick + ⅛" pegboard	(3)	.09	.35	1.17	.58	.24	.10	.60
3, 2" thick, unfaced		.22	.82	1.21	1.10	1.02	1.05	1.05
3, 2" thick + ¼" pegboard		.26	.97	1.12	.66	.34	.14	.75
3, 2" thick + perforated metal	(4)	.18	.73	1.14	1.06	.97	.93	1.00
3, 4" thick, unfaced		.84	1.24	1.24	1.08	1.00	.97	1.15
3, 4" thick + ¼" pegboard		.80	1.19	1.00	.71	.38	.13	.80
3, 6" thick, unfaced		1.09	1.15	1.13	1.05	1.04	1.04	1.10
3, 6" thick + ¼" pegboard		.95	1.04	.98	.69	.36	.18	.75

Table I-12, Sound absorption coefficients of fiberglass boards covered with various facings.
(1) Absorption values would be unchanged for open facings such as wire mesh, metal lath, or porous fabric.
(2) Perforated with ¼" holes, 1" on centers.
(3) Perforated with ⅛" holes, 1" on centers.
(4) 24 gauge, ³⁄₃₂" holes, 13% open area.

Product Type & Thickness	OCTAVE BAND CENTER FREQUENCIES, Hz						
	125	250	500	1000	2000	4000	NRC
Brick, unglazed	.03	.03	.03	.04	.05	.07	.05
Brick, unglazed, painted	.01	.01	.02	.02	.02	.03	.00
Concete block, painted	.10	.05	.06	.07	.09	.08	.05
Carpet, ⅛" pile height	.05	.05	.10	.20	.30	.40	.15
Carpet, ¼" pile height	.05	.10	.15	.30	.50	.55	.25
Carpet, ³⁄₁₆" combined pile and foam	.05	.10	.10	.30	.40	.50	.25
Carpet, ⁵⁄₁₆" combined pile and foam	.05	.15	.30	.40	.50	.60	.35
Fabric, light velour, 10 oz/sq. yd. hung straight in contact with wall	.03	.04	.11	.17	.24	.35	.15
Fabric, medium velour, 14 oz/sq. yd. draped to half area	.07	.31	.49	.75	.70	.60	.55
Fabric, heavy velour, 18 oz/sq. yd. draped to half area	.14	.35	.55	.72	.70	.65	.60
Floors, concrete or terrazzo	.01	.01	.01	.02	.02	.02	.00
Floors, linoleum, asphalt, rubber or cork tile on concrete	.02	.03	.03	.03	.03	.02	.05
Floors, wood	.15	.11	.10	.07	.06	.07	.10
Floors, wood parquet in asphalt or concrete	.04	.04	.07	.06	.06	.07	.05
Glass, ¼", sealed, large panes	.05	.03	.02	.02	.03	.02	.05
Glass, 24 oz. operable windows, closed	.10	.05	.04	.03	.03	.03	.05
Gypsum board, ½", nailed to 2x4s 16" on centers, painted	.10	.08	.05	.03	.03	.03	.05
Marble or glazed tile	.01	.01	.01	.01	.02	.02	.00
Plaster, gypsum or lime, rough finish or lath	.02	.03	.04	.05	.04	.03	.05
Plaster, gypsum or lime, smooth finish	.02	.02	.03	.04	.04	.03	.05
Hardwood plywood paneling, ¼" thick, wood frame	.58	.22	.07	.04	.03	.07	.10
Water surface, as in swimming pool	.01	.01	.01	.01	.02	.03	.00
Wood roof decking, tongue-and-groove cedar	.24	.19	.14	.08	.13	.10	.15

Above from *Acoustical Ceilings—Use and Practice*, Ceilings and Interior Systems Contractors Association (1984), p. 18.

Table I-13. Sound absorption coefficients of general building materials.

Section II - SOUND TRANSMISSION LOSS OF MATERIALS AND SYSTEMS:

Notes to Section II data:

(1) All tests were conducted according to ASTM E-90, Standard Method for Laboratory Measurement of Airborne Sound Transmission Loss of Building Partitions. The Transmission loss for each sample was measured over one- third-octave bands in order to determine a single number Sound Transmission Class (STC) rating. Transmission loss data are reported at the preferred octave band center frequencies.

(2) Sound insertion loss data in these tables are the difference between sound pressure levels measured at the center of a two foot square opening in the wall of a reverberation chamber excited by sound before and after a material is inserted in the opening.

(3) The surface weight of each material in pounds per square foot has been listed. Materials weighing the same as these materials can be expected to provide generally similar results.

Product Type & Thickness	OCTAVE BAND CENTER FREQUENCIES, Hz						NIC
	125	250	500	1000	2000	4000	
Plywood, ½", 1.33 lb/sq. ft. (3)	17	20	23	23	23	24	21
Plywood, ¾", 2.00 lb/sq. ft.	19	23	27	25	22	30	24
Sheet metal, 16 gauge, 2.38 lb/sq. ft.	18	22	28	31	35	41	31
Sheet metal, 20 gauge, 1.50 lb/sq. ft.	16	19	25	27	32	39	27
Sheet metal, 24 gauge, 1.02 lb/sq. ft.	13	16	23	24	29	36	25
Gypsum board, ½", 1.80 lb/sq. ft.	18	22	26	29	27	26	26
Gypsum board, ⅝", 2.20 lb/sq. ft.	19	22	25	28	22	31	26
Glass, single strength, 3/32", 1.08 lb/sq. ft.	15	18	25	26	28	29	26
Glass, double strength, ⅛", 1.40 lb/sq. ft.	16	19	25	29	30	20	24
Glass, plate, ¼", 2.78 lb/sq. ft.	20	25	26	30	23	30	27
Acrylic sheet, ⅛", 0.75 lb/sq. ft.	14	17	22	24	27	34	24
Acrylic sheet, ¼", 1.45 lb/sq. ft.	16	19	26	27	30	29	27
Acrylic sheet, ½", 2.75 lb/sq. ft.	20	24	27	30	29	35	29
Lead vinyl, 1.25 lb/sq. ft.	17	19	28	30	34	39	29

Table II-1. Sound Insertion Loss, of typical building materials.

Product Type & Thickness	\multicolumn{7}{c}{OCTAVE BAND CENTER FREQUENCIES, Hz}
	125	250	500	1000	2000	4000	NIC
FRP, ⅛" thick, 1.13 lb/sq. ft. (3)	15	18	25	26	29	36	27
FRP, ¼" thick, 2.08 lb/sq. ft.	19	22	28	31	32	25	29
FRP, ½" thick, 4.20 lb/sq.ft.	21	27	29	34	27	36	29

Table II-2. Sound Insertion Loss of Fibrous Glass Reinforced Plastics (FRP).

Construction Type	OCTAVE BAND CENTER FREQUENCIES, Hz						
	125	250	500	1000	2000	4000	NIC
Plywood enclosure, ½", unlined	13	11	12	12	13	15	13
Plywood enclosure, ½", lined with 703 insulation 1" thick	18	17	23	30	38	40+	28
Plywood enclosure, ½", lined with 703 insulation 2" thick	18	23	30	37	45	50+	34
Plywood enclosure, ½", lined with 703 insulation 4" thick	19	29	38	47	58	60+	39
Plywood enclosure, ½", lined with 3⅝" (R-13) insulation	17	25	29	36	41	45+	34

Table II-3. Sound Insertion Loss of plywood enclosures.

Construction Type	OCTAVE BAND CENTER FREQUENCIES, Hz						
	125	250	500	1000	2000	4000	STC
Metal building wall, 26 gauge	12	14	15	21	21	25	20
Metal building wall + 2" insulation	11	15	16	29	31	37	24
Metal building wall + 3" insulation	12	16	18	31	32	39	25

Table II-4, Sound transmission loss of metal building walls.

Construction Type	\multicolumn{6}{c}{OCTAVE BAND CENTER FREQUENCIES, Hz}	
	125	250	500	1000	2000	4000	NIC
Lead vinyl, 1.25 lb/sq. ft. + 2½" air space + lead vinyl, 1.25 lb/sq. ft.	12	34	31	37	43	48	34
Lead vinyl, 1.25 lb/sq. ft. + 2½" Fiberglas (R-8) insulation batt + lead vinyl, 1.25 lb/sq. ft.	25	34	38	43	47	58	42
Sheet metal, 16 gauge + 2½" air space + sheet metal, 16 gauge	23	33	34	37	38	48	37
Sheet metal, 16 gauge + 2½" Fiberglas (R-8) insulation batt + sheet metal, 16 gauge	26	33	36	38	41	51	38
Sheet metal, 16 gauge + 2½" Fiberglas (R-8) insulation batt + sheet metal, 24 gauge	20	36	37	41	44	52	40
Sheet metal, 20 gauge + 1" Fiberglas 475 duct board	18	17	30	38	47	55	32
Sheet metal, 20 gauge + 2 layers of 1" Fiberglas 475 duct board	15	18	35	42	51	56	32
Sheet metal, 20 gauge + 3 layers of 1" Fiberglas 475 duct board	16	23	40	46	52	61	31
Sheet metal, 16 gauge + 4½" Insul-Quick® insulation + 0.040" aluminum, 4" ribbed	31	45	48	58	64	64	50
Sheet metal, 16 gauge + 4½" TIW Type II insulation + 0.040" aluminum, 4" ribbed	25	43	48	56	63	61	48
703 insulation, plain, two 1" layers	7	6	5	10	16	20	11
703 insulation, FRK faced, two 1" layers, back to back	9	10	7	15	23	31	14

Table II-5. Sound Insertion Loss for special constructions.

Exterior finish	Cavity insulation	Resilient channel	STC
Wood siding	None	no	37
Wood siding	3½" (R-11) Fiberglas insulation	no	39
Wood siding	Reflective foil	no	37
Wood siding	3" (R-11) rock wool	no	38
Wood siding	None	yes	43
Wood siding	3½" (R-11) Fiberglas insulation	yes	47
Stucco	3½" (R-11) Fiberglas insulation	no	46
Stucco	None	yes	49
Stucco	3½" (R-11) Fiberglas insulation	yes	57
Brick veneer	3½" (R-11) Fiberglas insulation	no	56
Brick veneer	None	yes	54
Brick veneer	3½" (R-11) Fiberglas insulation	yes	58
Concrete block	None	no	45

Table II-6. Sound Transmission Loss for exterior wall constructions.

Construction Type	__OCTAVE BAND CENTER FREQUENCIES, Hz__						
	125	250	500	1000	2000	4000	STC
2½" metal studs, 24" centers, ½" gypsum wallboard both sides	13	21	33	43	44	39	34
2½" metal studs, 24" centers, ½" gypsum wallboard both sides + 2½" (R-8) Fiberglas insulation	22	33	44	51	52	43	42
2½" metal studs, 24" centers, 2 layers ½" gypsum wallboard both sides	23	30	45	49	52	52	45
2½" metal studs, 24" centers, 2 layers ½" gypsum wallboard one side, 1 layer ½" gypsum wallboard other side + 2½" (R-8) Fiberglas insulation	30	42	51	59	62	51	50
2½" metal studs, 24" centers, 2 layers ½" gypsum wallboard both sides + 2½" (R-8) Fiberglas insulation	36	45	54	62	65	56	54
3⅝" metal studs, 24" centers, ½" gypsum wallboard both sides	16	23	37	45	46	37	36
3⅝" metal studs, 24" centers, ½" gypsum wallboard both sides + 3½" (R-11) Fiberglas insulation	24	35	47	54	57	42	44
3⅝" metal studs, 24" centers, 2 layers ½" gypsum wallboard one side, 1 layer ½" gypsum wallboard other side	21	29	43	50	51	42	41
3⅝" metal studs, 24" centers, 2 layers ½" gypsum wallboard one side, 1 layer ½" gypsum wallboard other side, + 3½" (R-11) Fiberglas insulation	33	44	52	60	63	53	52
3⅝" metal studs, 24" centers, 2 layers ½" gypsum wallboard both sides	30	40	49	55	58	52	50
3⅝" metal studs, 24" centers, 2 layers ½" gypsum wallboard both sides + 3½" (R-11) Fiberglas insulation	38	47	55	58	63	57	56

Table II-7. Sound Transmission Loss for metal stud wall constructions.

Door Type	Weather Strip	Normally Closed STC
Wood, flush solid core, 1¾", 3.9 lb/sq.ft.	Brass	27
Wood, flush solid core, 1¾", 3.9 lb/sq.ft.	Plastic	27
Steel, flush, 1¾", 3.2 lb/sq.ft., 0.028" steel faces separated by plastic perimeter strip, with rigid polyurethane foam core, 2 to 2.5 lb/cu.ft., foamed in place	Magnetic	28

Table II-8. Sound Transmission Loss for exterior doors.

Construction Type	\multicolumn{6}{c}{OCTAVE BAND CENTER FREQUENCIES, Hz}	
	125	250	500	1000	2000	4000	STC
2"x4" wood studs, 16" centers, ½" gypsum wallboard both sides	15	27	36	42	47	40	35
2"x4" wood studs, 16" centers, ½" gypsum wallboard both sides + 3½" (R-11) Fiberglas insulation	15	31	40	46	50	42	39
2"x4" wood studs, 16" centers, 2 layers of ½" gypsum wallboard one side, 1 layer of ½" gypsum wallboard other side	17	32	40	45	50	45	38
2"x4" wood studs, 16" centers, 2 layers of ½" gypsum wallboard both sides	15	35	43	48	53	50	39
2"x4" wood studs, 16" centers, 2 layers of ½" gypsum wallboard both sides + 3½" (R-11) Fiberglas insulation	21	37	45	50	55	51	45
2"x4" wood studs, 16" centers, resilient channel one side, ½" gypsum wallboard both sides	15	32	40	49	52	45	39
2"x4" wood studs, 16" centers, resilient channel one side, ½" gypsum wallboard both sides + 3½" (R-11) Fiberglas insulation	22	40	53	57	58	50	46
2"x4" wood studs, staggered construction, 24" centers, ½" gypsum wallboard both sides	22	23	36	46	52	41	38
2"x4" wood studs, staggered construction, 24" centers, ½" gypsum wallboard both sides + 3½" (R-11) Fiberglas insulation	31	37	47	52	56	50	49
2"x4" wood studs, 24" centers, double stud construction, ½" gypsum wallboard both sides	21	33	43	47	47	44	41
2"x4" wood studs, 24" centers, double stud construction, ½" gypsum wallboard both sides + 3½" (R-11) Fiberglas insulation	33	46	58	63	64	61	56
2"x4" wood studs, 24" centers, double stud construction, 2 layers ½" gypsum wallboard both sides + 3½" (R-11) Fiberglas insulation	44	55	63	67	71	71	64

Table II-9, Sound Transmission Loss for wood stud wall constructions.

Material	Type	Size	Glazing*	Sealed STC	Locked STC	Unlocked STC
Wood	Double hung	3'x5'	ss	29		23
Wood	Double hung	3'x5'	ss/dl	29		
Wood	Double hung	3'x5'	ds	29		
Wood	Double hung	3'x5'	ds/dl	30		
Wood	Double hung	3'x5'	ins 7/16"	28	26	22
Wood	Fixed picture	6'x5'	ss/dl	28		
Wood	Fixed picture	6'x5'	ds	29		
Wood	Fixed picture	6'x5'	ins 1"	34		
Wood/Plastic	Double hung	3'x5'	ss	29	26	26
Wood/Plastic	Double hung	3'x5'	ins 3/8"	26	26	25
Wood/Plastic	storm sash	3'x5'	ds	30	27	
Wood/Plastic	storm sash	3'x5'	ins 3/8"	28	24	
Wood/Plastic	Fixed casement	3'x5'	ds	31		
Wood/Plastic	Operable casement	3'x5'	ds		30	22
Wood/Plastic	Sliding		lam 3/16"	31	26	26
Aluminum	Sliding		ss	28	24	
Aluminum	Operable casement		ds	31	21	17
Aluminum	Single hung		ins 7/16"	30	27	25
Single pane 1/4" laminated glass						34

Table II-10. Sound Transmission Loss for windows.

Data from U.S. Department of Commerce National Bureau of Standards Building Science Series 77.
*Abbreviations: ss = single strength
ds = double strength   ins = insulated (overall thickness indicated)
dl = divided lights   lam = laminated (overall thickness indicated)

NOTES TO TABLES, SECTION II,

(1) All tests were conducted according to ASTM C 423, Standard Test Method for Sound Absorption and Sound Absorption Coefficients by the Reverberation Room Method. NIC and STC ratings for each sample were measured over one-third octave bands and are reported at the preferred octave band center frequencies.

(2) The sound insertion loss data in these tables are the difference between sound pressure levels measured at the center of a 2 foot square opening in the wall of a reverberation chamber excited by sound before and after a material is inserted in the opening.

(3) The surface weight of each material in pounds per square foot has been listed. Materials weighing the same as these materials can be expected to provide generally similar results.

Acoustical Data   155

Section III - DUCT AND DUCT LINER MATERIALS

This information was provided by Owens Corning Fiberglas. Similar results may be expected by competitive materials. Check with manufacturer for actual values.

Notes to Section III:

(1) Tested at air velocity of 2000 feet per minute. Attenuation data for duct liners are based on sound pressure levels measured in a reverberation room after sound passes through a 10 foot specimen and enters the reverberation room. These tests were conducted according to ASTM Method E 477. Attenuation data for other duct systems may differ from these values, and may be higher or lower depending on the distribution of sound energy in various propagating duct modes, length of lined (or unlined) duct sections (which create discontinuities in the boundary conditions along the perimeter) and exit conditions at duct terminations.

* P/A: The inside perimeter of a lined duct in feet divided by the cross sectional free area of the duct in square feet.

P/A = 3 is based on a 12" x 24" duct
P/A = 4 is based on a 12" x 12" duct
P/A = 5 is based on a 8" x 8" duct
P/A = 6 is based on a 6" x 12" duct
P/A = 7 is based on a 6" x 6" duct

APPENDIX 4

Product	P/A*	OCTAVE BAND CENTER FREQUENCIES, Hz					
		125	250	500	1000	2000	4000
Aeroflex® duct liner, Type 150, 1" thick	3	0.5	0.5	1.5	2.8	4.0	2.7
	4	0.6	0.8	2.0	3.4	3.9	3.6
	5	0.5	1.2	2.1	3.4	5.1	3.8
	6	0.2	1.1	2.4	3.5	3.9	3.7
	8	0.4	1.7	3.1	4.0	4.8	4.4
Aeroflex duct liner, Type 150, 2" thick	3	0.9	1.1	3.2	4.6	3.5	2.6
	4	0.9	1.5	3.0	4.1	3.9	3.8
	5	0.5	1.8	3.4	4.7	5.3	4.1
	6	0.4	1.3	3.1	3.6	3.9	3.5
	8	0.4	1.8	3.7	4.2	4.8	4.4
Aeroflex duct liner, Type 200, 1" thick	3	0.7	0.6	1.7	2.9	4.1	2.8
	4	0.6	0.7	2.0	3.4	4.1	3.7
	5	0.2	1.1	2.1	3.5	5.3	3.8
	6	0.3	1.0	2.4	3.4	3.8	3.4
	8	0.4	1.7	2.9	3.9	4.6	4.4
Duct liner board, 1" thick	3	0.4	0.5	1.7	4.4	3.8	2.2
	6	0.3	0.9	2.7	4.7	5.2	4.1
Duct liner board, 2" thick	3	0.6	1.0	3.8	4.7	3.6	2.3
	6	0.4	2.0	4.1	4.7	5.1	3.7

Table III-1. Duct attenuation in dB per lineal foot of fiberglass duct liner.

Product	P/A*	OCTAVE BAND CENTER FREQUENCIES, Hz					
		125	250	500	1000	2000	4000
Aeroflex® duct liner, Type 150, 1" thick	3	10	14	20	25	31	32
	4	10	13	26	29	34	35
	5	5	13	22	26	30	31
	6	2	11	22	26	32	33
	8	2	10	14	20	24	29
Aeroflex duct liner, Type 150, 2" thick	3	13	16	24	30	36	37
	4	12	15	27	31	34	36
	5	7	17	24	26	30	33
	6	5	14	26	28	31	34
	8	3	11	16	20	25	28
Aeroflex duct liner, Type 200, 1" thick	3	10	13	23	28	30	27
	4	10	13	26	30	34	36
	5	4	14	24	27	30	32
	6	2	14	24	27	30	32
	8	2	14	19	25	29	34
Duct liner board, 1" thick	3	9	13	24	25	30	35
	6	4	16	26	30	33	36
Duct liner board, 2" thick	3	12	17	28	30	37	42
	6	4	16	23	28	33	34

Table III-2. Radiated noise reduction in dB for ducts lined with duct liner (similar to single pass transmission loss through duct sidewall)

****

Appendix 5 - BIBLIOGRAPHY

Bell, L. H. *Fundamentals of Industrial Noise Control.*
        Trumbull, CT: Harmony, 1973.
Bell, L. H. *Industrial Noise Control*
        New York, NY: Marcel Dekker, 1982.
Broch, J. T. *Mechanical Vibrations and Shock Measurements*
        Marlborough, Massachusetts: Bruel and Kjaer
Beranek, L. L. *Acoustic Measurements*
        New York, NY: Wiley, 1949
Beranek, L. L. *Acoustics*
        New York, NY: McGraw-Hill, 1954
Beranek, L. L. *Noise and Vibration Control*
        New York, NY: McGraw-Hill, 1971
Brendt, R. D. and E. L. R. Corliss, E.L.R. *Quieting: A Practical Guide to Noise Control*
        Washington, DC: National Bureau of Standards, 1976
Crede, C. E. *Vibration and Shock Isolation*
        New York, NY: Wiley, 1951
Egan, D. M. *Concepts in Architectural Acoustics*
        New York, NY: McGraw-Hill, 1972
Faulkner, L. *Handbook of Industrial Noise Control*
        New York, NY: Industrial Press, 1975
Harris, C. M. *Handbook of Noise Control*
        New York, NY: McGraw-Hill, 1957
Harris, C. M. and C. E. Crede *Shock and Vibration Handbook*
        New York, NY: McGraw-Hill, 1961
Harris, D. A., et al *Planning and Designing the Office Environment*
        New York, NY: Van Nostrand Reinhold, 1981
                - 2nd edition (expanded) 1991.
Jens, T. B. *Acoustic Noise Measurements*
        Marlborough, Massachusetts: Bruel and Kjaer, 1971
Irwin, J. D. and E. R. Graf *Industrial Noise and Vibration Control*
        Englewood Cliffs, NJ: Prentice-Hall,1979
Kinsler, L. E. and A. R. Frey *Fundamentals of Acoustics*
        New York, NY: Wiley, 1950
Morse, P. M. *Vibration and Sound, 1st ed.* 1936
Morse, P. M. and K. U. Ingard *Theoretical Acoustics*
        New York, NY: McGraw-Hill, 1968
Harris, D. A. *Noise Control Manual* Pub. #5-BMG-8277-G
        Toledo, OH: Owens Corning Fiberglas, 1986

Peterson, A.P. and E. E. Gross Jr. *E.E. Handbook of Noise Measurement*
        Concord, MA,: GenRad, 1972
Purcell, W. E. *Systems for Noise and Vibration Control*
        Westlake, OH: Sound and Vibration Magazine, August 1982.
Purcell, W. E. *Materials for Noise Control*
        Westlake, OH: Sound and Vibration Magazine, July, 1982

****

INDEX

Acoustical Data 141-156
    Sound Absorbing Materials 141
    Sound Transmission Loss of Materials and Systems 149
        Partitions, Floor/Ceilings, Exterior Walls, Doors, Windows
    Duct and Duct Liner Materials 155
acoustical material 5, 95, 97, 105
Acoustical Standards Appendix 2, 101, 106, 118
    ASTM, ISO, ASHRAE, ANSI, IEEE, NCA, NEMA, SAE, IEC and others
airborne sound 23, 28, 32, 70, 71, **95-99, 108-110**, 112, 116, 149
Airflow-Generated Sound Power Levels 115
ambient noise 95
Application Standards 113
Articulation Class (AC) 81, 86, 92, 93, 106-108
ASTM Committee E33, Environmental Acoustics, Appendix 2, 102
average sound pressure level 95, 132
Average Sound Level (L) 110
Average Insertion Loss 116
background noise 23, 95, 111
Bibliography 157
building facade 14, 19, 26, 27, 31, 32, 64, 69, 70, 73, 76, 88, 89, 92, 96, 97, 99, 104-106, **108-112**, 115, 126, 127, **130-133**, 136, 138, 139, 141, 142, 144, 146, 149, 150
Community Noise Standards 117
composite loss factor 36, 43, 95
damp 35, 95, 20
decay rate 15, 36, 95
decibel (dB) 95
Design Guide and Worksheets 119-140
    Calculating A weighted Sound Levels 119
    Reverberant Sound Control Guidelines 121
    Examples of SPR (Source/Path/Receiver) Noise Control 124
    Controlling Environmental Noise 132
    Determining the Sound Transmission Loss of a Composite Partition 133
    Controlling Noise Within Plant Boundaries 136
    Controlling Noise in Adjacent Office Areas 136
    Noise Reduction Within a Room 137
    Community Noise and Other Noise 137
diffraction 126
diffraction 13, 74, 95
diffuse sound field 96, 98, 99
direct sound field 96

Environmental Protection Agency (EPA) 3
field transmission loss (FTL) 109
field sound transmission class (FSTC) 96, 109
Field Impact Insulation Class (FLIC) 112
flanking transmission 7, 8, 17, 18, 28, 30, 69, 70, 72, 82, 83, **86-88**, 93, 94, 96, 108-110, 114, 136, 137
floor-ceiling assemblies 96, 112
Flow Ratio 116
Free Layer Damping Materials 40
frequency 1-5, 11-16, 18, 19, 24-27, 36, 37, 40-48, 50, 51, 64, 65, 68, 69, 77, 78, 92, 95-100, **103-106**, 109, 110, 112, 119, 121, 126-128, 132, 133
frequency band 5, 13, 15, 18, 69, 104, 132
Glossary of Acoustical Terms 95-100
insertion loss (IL) 96, 115
level (L) 96, 110
level reduction (LR) 96
Mechanical and Electrical System Noise Standards 115
metric sabin [L2] 97
noise reduction (NR) 34, 97, 109, 111
noise isolation class (NIC) 109-111
noise reduction class (NRC) 82
noise isolation class (NIC) 97
Noise Control Association (NCA) Acknowledgements, 50, 90
Noise Control Technology 1, 10
    What is Noise? 1
    Measurement of Sound 2
    Noise Exposure Levels (OSHA) 3
    Basic Principals of Noise Control 5
    Source Control 6
normal mode 97
normalized noise reduction (NNR) 97, 109
Normalized Sound Level Difference (Dn) 110
Normalized Impact Sound Pressure Levels (Ln) 112
Normalized Sound Level Difference (Dn) 110
Occupational Safety and Health Agency (OSHA) 3
Office Acoustics 67, **81, 83, 85, 84, 91, 93**, 107, 137
    Office Acoustics are Changing 81
    Challenge of the 90s 81
    The Sound of Silence 82
    Test Development 83
    Open Plan Product and Systems Solutions 86
        Ceilings, Part High Barriers, Vertical Surfaces, Masking,
    Closed/Open Design Dilemma 87
    Quiet Floors 89

       How to Specify 89
       Material and System Selection 89
       Standards for Open Plan Office 92
       Acoustical Criteria for Confidential Speech Privacy 94
Open Office Acoustical Standards 106
Outdoor-Indoor Transmission Loss (OITL) 97, 110, 111
Outdoor-Indoor Transmission Class (OITC) 76, 111
Outdoor-Indoor Level Reduction (OILR) 110
pink noise 97
pipe noise 34
pneumatic exhaust silencers 116
receiving room 23, 32, 71, 97, 109, 110, 112
reverberant sound field 97, 98, 121
reverberation 6, 15, 17, 22, 32, 48, 64, 66, 67, 82, 97, 99, **102-105**, 108, 109, 111, 115, 121, 126, 141, 149, 155
reverberation room 15, 17, 22, 48, 97, 98, 104, 111, 115, 141, 155
sabin [L2] 97
Silencers 9, 10, 33, 63, 73, 75, 80, **45-51**, 115, 116
       Silencer Types 45
       Active Duct Silencers 49

sound absorption 102
sound absorption coefficient (α) 98
Sound Absorbing Materials 6, 7, **9**, 45, 81, 82, 126, 136, 137, 141
       Material Types 9
       Sound Absorbing Materials (description) 10
       Sound Absorption Testing 15
       Specific Absorption Materials - Comments 18
Sound Absorption Standards 104
sound attenuation 7, 18, 34, **46-48, 69-71**, 74, 76, 78, 79, 82, 83, 98, 100, 108, 124, 127, 128
Sound Barrier Materials/Systems 23
       Sound Barrier Function 23
       Sound Transmission Loss 24
       Specific Barrier Materials 27
       Barrier Systems 30
       Test Procedures for Sound Transmission Loss 32
       Duct Attenuation 32
       Pipe Noise 34
sound insulation 109
sound isolation 73, 93, 97, 98, 107, 110
sound intensity 98
sound leaks 7, 8, 30, 72, 75, 76, 78, 86, 87, 114, 124, 130, 131, 136, 137
sound level 2, 3, 5, 15, 23, 71, 77, 82, 87, 93, 95, 98, 103, 110, 116, 117, 119, 124, 131, 138
Sound Level Difference (D) 110

sound pressure (p) 99
sound pressure level (Lp) 99
sound power (W) 99
sound power level (Lw) 99, 115
sound transmission class (STC) 22, 27, 31, 32, 70, 72, 82, 93, 99, **108, 109**, 149
sound transmission loss (TL) 99
Sound Transmission Standards 108
source room 71, 97, 99, 110, 111
speech privacy noise isolation class (NIC') 81, 84
speech privacy potential (SPP) 81, 84
structureborne sound 36, 100
Systems for Noise Control 63, 80
    System Types 63
    Sound Absorptive Systems 64
        Ceilings, Roof Decks and Exposed Floor Systems, Wall Treatments, Partitions, Functional Absorbers
    Sound Barrier Systems 69-80
        Ceilings, Floor/Ceiling Systems, Partition Systems, Demountable Partitions, Moveable Wall Systems, Sound Control Panels, Enclosures, Quiet Rooms, Pre-assembled Structures and Modules, Doors, Windows, Curtains, Pipe Lagging, Air Duct Systems
tapping machine 96, 70, 112, 113
vibration isolation 9, 10, 18, 35, **63**, 77, 100,
Vibration Isolation Materials 53
    Types of Vibration Isolation Materials 53
    Transmissibility and Damping 55
Vibration Damping Materials 35
    Damping vibrations 35
    Measuring Damping 36
    Types of Treatment 36
    Common Damping Materials 38
    Bonding 38
    Constrained Layer Materials 39
    Post Laminated Constrained Layer Systems 39
    Pre Laminated Metals 40
    Free Layer Damping Materials 40
white noise 100